**KT-238-403**

# Overcoming Common Problems Series

Overcoming Common Problems

# Sleep Better

## The science and the myths

PROFESSOR GRAHAM LAW
AND
DR SHANE PASCOE

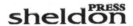

First published in Great Britain in 2017

Sheldon Press
36 Causton Street
London SW1P 4ST
www.sheldonpress.co.uk

*British Library Cataloguing-in-Publication Data*
A catalogue record for this book is available from the British Library

ISBN 978–1–84709–457–5
eBook ISBN 978–1–84709–458–2

Typeset by Fakenham Prepress Solutions, Fakenham, Norfolk NR21 8NN
First printed in Great Britain by Ashford Colour Press
Subsequently digitally printed in Great Britain

eBook by Fakenham Prepress Solutions, Fakenham, Norfolk NR21 8NN

Produced on paper from sustainable forests

# Contents

# Foreword

What skill or attribute are you most proud of? My talent is not immediately obvious, I don't look like a model and I cannot sing, but once I turn out the light I can sleep. I used to take this (apparently) simple thing for granted, although after 25 years' researching sleep and working with people who have sleep disorders, I have learned just how complex the process of falling asleep is and how much those with sleep disorders suffer. It has been estimated that sleep loss costs the UK economy over £40 billion per year, and is linked to two of the most important health epidemics in our society: obesity and dementia. There is no question about it: we need to learn how to sleep better and make time for this important activity.

I first met Graham a few years ago at a meeting of the British Sleep Society with several hundred sleep scientists, doctors and healthcare workers. Graham told me he wanted to understand the links between sleep and health, and I cannot think of a better person to do this. He is an outstanding scientist and one of the UK's leading sleep specialists. In this book he and Shane have done a great job exploring the myths about sleep, and by doing so have revealed facts and provided excellent top tips. For many the quest to sleep better includes drugs and alcohol, but Graham and Shane have looked further afield. Their book explains why laptops and clutter in the bedroom make our sleep worse, and even bananas – which I love, although luckily I eat them for breakfast (unlike Graham's mother-in-law).

This book contains much that I found thought-provoking. The authors' careful exploration has clearly shown that our sleep habits are learned early, probably in adolescence, and that good sleep is linked with better school grades. Since many adolescents experience a biological drive to go to bed and get up later (Chapter 26), there is now a public health debate about making school start times later. I am a night owl and hate getting up early, so I am all for later starts. I was also comforted to find I am not alone in this, and like Graham's wife and sister-in-law, I am a fan of the snooze button, although this is something Graham warns against for good sleep.

I really enjoyed the personal accounts in the book and am now also a fan of Graham's Gran, who appears in Chapter 20.

Perhaps the chapters with the most impact are those on mindfulness (Chapter 7) and the value of being an individual (Chapter 24). Graham and Shane emphasize that sleep is not a competition. We all need to sleep enough for our own needs. So whether you are a new parent, shift worker or, like me, have a long commute to work, this book has top tips for us all to stay healthy.

*Professor Mary Morrell, President of the British Sleep Society and*
*Professor of Sleep and Respiratory Physiology,*
*Imperial College, London*

# Welcome

Some clever people have said that it takes 10,000 hours' practice to become an expert at something. The Beatles and Bill Gates spent this long perfecting their music and computer programming. How is this relevant to you?

It is simple: by the age of three you have slept for at least 10,000 hours, so that makes you an expert at sleeping. So why is it, with all this expertise, that so many people have difficulty with their sleep? Our society is slowly beginning to recognize the issues we all have with sleep and how this affects our lives, health and well-being.

Do you have difficulty with your sleep? Are you reading this to try to find a 'solution'? When I tell people I am a sleep scientist, they often then tell me all about their sleep. (Incidentally, throughout this book 'I' refers to me, Graham, as I will be your guide. Shane will of course be offering his advice as a psychologist and practitioner of cognitive behavioural therapy for insomnia.) Usually they tell me their issues, sometimes their successes. In hearing about everyone's trials and tribulations, it struck me how many myths there are surrounding sleep. It never ceases to amaze me that after many years I still come across ones I've never heard before. Who would have thought that the full moon would affect your sleep? That's a new one I heard about in the process of writing this book. I won't deal with that myth here – after all, we have no control over the moon.

I find the whole subject of sleep fascinating, and humans have found it so for centuries, maybe millennia. Westernized societies have fairy tales based on sleep: Sleeping Beauty, the Princess and the Pea, Rip Van Winkle. This book is going to explore myths surrounding sleep. Some of these myths are informative and helpful, some incorrect and some positively damaging and counterproductive.

Shane uses cognitive behavioural therapy for insomnia (CBTi), which is often prescribed or recommended to deal with sleep disorders, and the method we are using in this book has some similarities. We have split the issues people have into small, self-contained subjects. It is very common for people to consider sleep to be a single entity, with a single issue. That is far from the truth.

In fact there are many issues, all interconnected. We will work through each of these myths to see which are unhelpful and which may be worth taking further and might help you deal with any sleep issues.

This book will look at how our current knowledge can be used to improve your sleep. This will require some work on your part. I am very sceptical of a simple 'cure', a tablet or a diet, a basic method. These probably will not work. The reality is that solving sleep issues is difficult, time-consuming and hard work. You will need to be dedicated, careful and thoughtful.

In this book you will read about a number of ways to approach different types of difficulties with sleep. Each chapter is a stand-alone entity and they don't need to be read in any particular order. The final chapter will summarize what we know at the moment and how science can help you sleep better.

# 1

# 'I should have 8 hours' sleep'

Barack Obama was asked what he would like most for Christmas after a year of campaigning to be president of the United States. He answered without hesitation: 'Eight hours' sleep.'

When I ask people what they know about sleep, the first answer is nearly always: 'You need 8 hours.' We are going to look at the evidence in support of this myth and how this belief can influence your sleep. The media promotes it, and you see it in books and on television. Of course, most of you will know of somebody who says they don't require a full 8 hours. There are reports of the late Margaret Thatcher only needing 4 hours' sleep per night; people wear the ability to survive on a limited amount of sleep as a badge of honour. The politically convenient perception was that she was tough, the 'Iron Lady', and 8 hours was therefore for weaker people, but is this true? Does everyone need 8 hours? Is everyone the same?

## The myth came from medical research

As this myth seems to be widely quoted, where did it originate? During the 1980s and 1990s there was a group of scientists, led by Thomas Wehr in Washington DC, who were interested in the length of time humans sleep. One particular experiment they carried out – in which I would not like to have been a 'guinea pig' – made eight people live in rooms where they were only allowed 10 hours' light per day. It was pitch-black for the other 14 hours, and they were not permitted to listen to music or have anything that might interrupt their sleep patterns.

To begin with, these people slept an average of 11 hours per night. The reason for sleeping 11 hours may have been because they were catching up on a sleep 'debt' that had built up. After 4 weeks, seven of the participants were sleeping for around 8 hours, broken into two blocks of around 4 hours. Adding these two blocks together has led to the idea that we need 8 hours' sleep per night.

Surveys over the past few decades have also supported the need for 8 hours per night. The overwhelming majority say that people have an average of 7–8 hours' sleep per night. By looking at some of the national and international surveys, we can get a clear picture of what is a standard or an average amount of sleep. A study I have worked on as part of my research, known as Understanding Society, shows that adults in the UK sleep on average 7 hours and 10 minutes. However, this is an average and the number of hours of sleep varies hugely between individuals – from 3.5 hours to 11 hours or more. Some 10 per cent of people report having more than 10 hours' sleep per night, and over one-third say they sleep fewer than 7 hours. It is clear that the eight-hour myth hides significant variation – and an experiment with only eight people will not tell the whole story.

## How much sleep do you need?

So how much do we need? It seems we are all different – 'Nowt as queer as folk' you might say. When Napoleon Bonaparte was asked how many hours' sleep people need, he replied 'Six for a man, seven for a woman, eight for a fool.'

This is one of the most valuable and insightful phrases about the amount of sleep you should have. It shows a disregard for personal differences and the events happening around you in your lives when you try to sleep. Do you believe that the stronger a person is perceived to be, the less sleep they need?

You need to ignore these implied, and sometimes explicit, stereotypes. Each person needs different amounts of sleep. These differences may be due to your genetic composition, lifestyle and levels of activity, health or other factors; also, these needs change for the same person as they get older or during particular phases of life that they experience.

The key to understanding whether or not you have had enough sleep is noticing if there is excessive sleepiness, particularly during the daytime. Sometimes people report very little sleep but have no excessive daytime sleepiness. Therefore it is reasonably straightforward to ascertain that they have in fact had 'enough' sleep.

The idea of stating an amount of time you need to sleep is similar to stating the number of calories you should consume. It is well understood that different people need different amounts of energy. The calorie intake differs with age and by sex. During times when you are doing large amounts of exercise, your body needs more energy, but when you are trying to gain or lose weight, there is a different requirement. Also, some people simply need more than others to maintain a constant weight.

Individual differences are also present for sleep. So why should someone say 'Everyone needs 8 hours' sleep'? We risk oversimplifying a complex issue, and maybe you could give them an alternative viewpoint.

## Summary

The evidence shows that there is some truth in this myth: the average time a population of people sleep for is around 8 hours, and some individuals will need 8 hours' sleep. This 'average' is not necessarily you, though. We do not all weigh an 'average' weight or own a house with the 'average' house price. As an individual you will have your own requirement, and it is important to work out what that is for you, rather than try to achieve the average amount, which may be too much or too little for you.

## Top tips

1 Work out how much sleep you need. A good way to start is to keep a sleep diary for a couple of weeks. There are many available online – search 'sleep diary'. An industry standard is the American Academy of Sleep Medicine's sleep diary (visit <http://yoursleep.aasmnet.org/pdf/sleepdiary.pdf>). Filling this in for a couple of weeks should give you an idea of how you are sleeping at the moment. It would be good to repeat this as you work your way through this book. The tips in each chapter will help you improve your sleep, and you should see this reflected in your sleep diary.

2 When you have a day on which you wake feeling refreshed and do not feel excessively sleepy through the day, the sleep you had is the right amount for you.

3 Do not allow yourself to be convinced by others that there is a 'right' amount of sleep. It doesn't matter what your friends do or tell you – only you can know what is right for you.

# 2

# 'You lose weight by sleeping less'

This myth comes about because of our society's view of sloth: one of the 'seven deadly sins', seen as a completely negative behaviour and attitude. Although a single definition of this sin is difficult, the most common one revolves around laziness. How about thinking for a moment how you would represent laziness? You probably imagine someone very overweight and either lying down or asleep. So you can see how we have conflated these two different issues: weight and sleep.

Confused thinking, usually in the form of logical errors, is how myths arise and there are some who think that oversleeping leads to weight gain. Therefore, in reverse, it would seem to make sense that if you sleep less, you will lose weight, but the opposite is correct. People who lack sleep will often, on average, be more overweight. Overall, a good sleep pattern with at least 6 hours' sleep could lead to a weight loss of 4.5 kilograms (a little under 10 pounds), according to well-conducted scientific trials.

## Lack of sleep leads to weight gain

There are a number of reasons why sleeping too little leads to gaining weight. The first relates to tiredness during the daytime. When you feel tired you may choose to drink coffee or a sweet drink. I certainly do that, and when I feel extravagant I will choose a mocha – coffee and chocolate mixed, with a little sugar. This is intended to make you feel livelier, more awake. A further tempta-tion you may have given into is to have a snack: a biscuit, a small piece of chocolate, a wafer-thin mint, a piece of the office cake.

It is common for people to eat to feel better, which is known as emotional eating. A lack of sleep causes your body to crave happy feelings. Your brain's reward centres light up and crave more rewards. Easy rewards are fat-laden, and sugary, foods and drinks. This is well understood as a style of consumption that can lead to weight gain. There is also an unwanted spiral here. Increasing weight can lead to negative feelings, which in turn lead to a poorer quality of sleep – and so the cycle repeats.

The daytime tiredness will also lead to your having less energy and lower motivation to exercise. Your weight is the result of energy in, through food and drink, and energy out, which includes exercise. If you use less energy because you are too tired to exercise, this leads to a potential for weight gain. Exercise is also a good way to improve the quality of your sleep and your ability to fall asleep. This is another vicious circle: less exercise leads to poorer sleep, which leads to less exercise.

The second reason why sleeping too little leads to weight gain has been explored in clinical trials, which are the best studies that medical science can perform. In one of these, a group of people were asked to go to bed much later than was normal for them, which led to their having a mere 4 hours' sleep per night. When this group was compared with a group of people who slept normally, the results were amazing: those in the sleep-deprived group had put on weight. This was probably because there was more time in their day: an extra 3 or 4 hours. How did they fill the time? Especially when we are feeling very tired, we eat; and we eat those foods that are crunchy on the outside and soft on the inside, which is the best way to describe the most fattening foods: doughnuts, sausages, cakes, fried potatoes and so on. The group also chose larger portions than they would normally have during the day.

A third reason, partly related to the sleep loss, is hormonal. The key hormones here are called ghrelin and leptin. Ghrelin tells your body when it is ready to eat. It is the 'go' hormone and leptin is the 'stop' hormone. With the release of leptin your body feels full and no longer wants to eat. Research suggests that sleep deprivation leads to more ghrelin, therefore you want to eat more, and less leptin, which makes you less likely to stop eating.

The reverse of this relationship between food and sleep also leads to poor sleep. For example, large meals, close to bedtime, are likely to cause you to have an interrupted sleep. This will then go back into the pattern of eating more and sleeping less. Finally, lack of sleep leads to you not focusing properly, not taking sufficient care of yourself. Then that strict diet you may have adopted can soon go wrong because you are not awake enough to have any self-discipline.

## Summary

Despite what some people think, sufficient sleep may help you to control your weight. When your sleep is out of control, this can lead to emotional eating and less motivation to exercise. Both of these are likely to lead to weight gain. The loss of focus and motivation may also make sticking to a diet and exercise plan more difficult.

## Top tips

1 Celebrate the fact that by improving your sleep you are also helping to control your weight. What a bonus!

2 Think carefully about your sleep patterns and how these may influence your weight management.

3 Try to avoid those vicious circles I talked about by maintaining your motivation for sticking with a sensible eating plan with regular exercise. Try looking at the NHS Choices website 'How to Diet' article at <www.nhs.uk/Livewell/loseweight/Pages/how-to-diet.aspx>. Also, Shane recommends knowing more about your personality and your individual behaviour when making changes. The Commonwealth Scientific and Industrial Research Organisation (CSIRO) has developed a 5-minute survey to help inform your diet choices – see <https://my.totalwellbeingdiet.com/Diet-Type>.

# 3

# 'I didn't sleep a wink last night'

Have you ever said 'I didn't sleep a wink last night'? Or have you heard anyone else say it? Of course, it might just be an exaggeration at times, but most people are fairly convinced they actually know how long they have slept.

How do you know how long you slept? You do know the time when you wake up. You glance at the clock or your mobile phone, or maybe your bed partner tells you. However, by definition you cannot know when you fall asleep, because, well, you are asleep. It sounds obvious but it doesn't stop people from claiming they know how long they have slept. Indeed, scientists, including myself, often ask people how long they sleep. When answering, they probably remember the time they last glanced at the clock while trying to fall asleep; then they probably subtract that from the sleep figure to give a length of time that they think it actually took to fall asleep.

There are now some ways to measure when you sleep. Modern technology, using what is known as an accelerometer, can measure times when you do not move. I use accelerometers in my research: small devices with a strap that you can wear on your wrist like a small digital watch. When I ask people to wear one, it looks a little as though they have been tagged by the prison service! The device attempts to define the time that you are asleep and uses different levels of sophistication. Using movement is not such a bad method, as for most people the first stages of sleep tend to involve a reduction in movement of the muscles.

You're probably thinking that sounds great for research, but isn't it expensive? It can be, but it is very likely that you already have an accelerometer, and I don't mean a prison tag. Most phones, certainly all smartphones, have a built-in accelerometer and this is what allows your device to know if it is moving and in which direction. There are also many 'apps' on smartphones that allow you to monitor your sleep and these use the built-in accelerometer. Of course, there is also an industry in wearable gadgets that measure movement.

Unfortunately, there remain difficulties in using these devices for measuring your sleep. When they are used to record the sleep of many thousands of people, they work well to estimate the average sleep time, but for an individual there are certain drawbacks. The risk lies in underestimating a young person's sleep and overestimating an older person's.

## Working out how long it takes you to fall asleep

So the measurement of sleep remains difficult. There is no clear cut-off between when you are asleep and when you are awake. It does not exist. Highly skilled sleep technicians can measure your brain activity and can determine that sleep has started. This uses complex technology which, fortunately, is beginning to reduce in price. One day this will be standard wearable technology, but until then you have to rely on your perceptions of sleep onset.

Research has been conducted into measuring when sleep starts. Early researchers, such as the 'sleep guru' Dr William Dement, founder of and emeritus professor at the Sleep Research Center at Stanford University, pioneered in 1977 a method known as the multiple sleep onset latency test. The aim was to work out how long it takes a person to fall asleep. If it takes less than 1 minute to nod off, this could indicate an underlying sleep disorder.

Dement and his colleagues realized that the more a person reports sleepiness, the quicker they will fall asleep. Making the link seems obvious, but it has been referred to as one of the most significant advances in the science of sleep. The test looked at a series of daytime naps and saw how many minutes it took a person to fall asleep – as simple as that.

Why am I telling you this? You do not have the clever machine they used, but you can do a home-based sleep-onset test developed by the physiologist and sleep researcher Nathaniel Kleitman. You lie in a quiet and dark room, comfortably, so that you could fall asleep. Place a plate on the floor and hold a spoon in your hand over the edge of the bed and make sure that if you let go of the spoon, it will hit the plate (but don't use your best china for this!).

Write down the time when you start to try to nap. Try to relax and fall asleep. Most people will nod off within 20 minutes or so. When you fall asleep, your hand will release the spoon and it will come crashing down on to the plate, waking you up. Immediately note down the time. The duration is the time elapsed between putting your head on the pillow and being woken by the noise of the spoon hitting the plate.

Dement warned against using this test in the evening, however, when you are naturally sleepier. When looking at your daytime nap, an elapsed time of 15 to 20 minutes indicates that you have no sleep debt. If you fall asleep within 5 minutes, you may have severe sleep deprivation.

## You may not be accurately assessing your sleep

Is there a single scientific test for sleepiness? Unfortunately, at the moment there is no such thing. It would revolutionize safety in this country, for example in factories operating heavy machinery, on the roads or in the aviation industry. A quick and, importantly, accurate test would be incredible. Some researchers have been looking at exactly this in fruit flies, which apparently do sleep. Who'd have known? A chemical called amylase increases in the fly saliva when they are sleep deprived, but it is very early days with this research and currently no test exists for humans.

Back to the idea that you think you didn't sleep at all. This thought is not an accurate description of what happened; it is usually an exaggeration. In a medical classification system known as the International Classification of Sleep Disorders, there is a documented disorder called paradoxical insomnia. The misperception involved arises when a person perceives himself to have remained awake when in fact he was asleep. The reverse may also happen, when someone reports sleeping when in fact she was awake. Scientists estimate that up to 5 per cent of people have this disorder at some level. There are no clearly understood causes, which also means that we have not identified ways to prevent it.

Advanced electrical monitoring machines, known as polysomnograms, have tested people with this disorder and demonstrated an overall regular pattern of sleep. However, sophisticated analysis of the patterns of brain activity does suggest that these people, often known as pseudo-insomniacs, have different patterns from those with healthy sleep. So we may be dealing with illusions of poor sleep or genuinely poor sleep due to a different brain activity. Either way, people with this disorder may have reduced feelings of well-being and difficulty maintaining a positive mood. There seems to be little treatment apart from the relief of symptoms through medication or behavioural or psychological intervention.

## Summary

You will probably have compared with other people the amount of sleep you have. It is a common question as part of normal conversation, and at first sight it seems simple to work out. This chapter has explained why this in fact remains a difficult question to answer.

## Top tips

1 Try the dropping-spoon method described above to see how long you take to fall asleep. As discussed, this is not an accurate assessment but can be fun!
2 Investigate the technology you already have on your smartphone if you have one. My experience is that people love gadgets that monitor their sleep. You could see what results you get over a period of time and use this alongside your sleep diary (see Chapter 1). As you read more of the book and discover techniques to improve your sleep, these measuring aids all help to monitor the effects of the changes you make.

# 4

# 'I'd be in trouble without my snooze button'

'I can't survive without my snooze button.'

Zoe Serrant, Graham's sister-in-law

The snooze button is a curiously problematic invention. The first snooze alarm clocks appeared in the 1950s. Lew Wallace, an American lawyer and author of the adventure tale *Ben-Hur: A tale of the Christ* (1880), is reported to have invented the snooze button, and presumably he thought it would be a great idea. However, it really goes against everything we know about sleep. As that statement may seem overly dramatic, it calls for an explanation.

Ask yourself: 'Why do I need my snooze button?' If you must wake at a certain time, then why not set your alarm for that time? It is because the snooze button gives you a different option. This option plays on two points: your love of a few minutes' more shuteye and your needing to get up and not be late. It is common for people to think that if they don't have a repeating alarm, then they will not get up.

The snooze button confuses the mind and body. You have been woken by an alarm, at which point the hormones in your body are being released to bring you to the point of being fully awake physically and mentally. This state of heightened alertness is important in an evolutionary sense in that historically we lived in a world where survival was paramount. When you tap the snooze mode, however, the body acts as if it is being allowed to return to a full sleep. You rest your head back on your pillow, curl up into your favourite sleep position. With this, your body resets all its hormones and prepares for sleep.

So what is the problem with this? The length of a standard sleep cycle is variable; it is different for different people and varies with age. Therefore it is difficult to be specific, but it is likely that a standard 10-minute snooze is too short for your body to feel rested again and ready to wake without that feeling of grogginess known as sleep inertia. This is while the mind makes the transition from sleeping to the fully awake mode. The amount of inertia experienced by people varies quite considerably, and probably leads to people regarding themselves as a 'morning person' (which is described as having low sleep inertia) or 'not a morning person'. Indeed, some recent research from the USA found that some people are so groggy that they have what is called sleep drunkenness, a serious deficit of ability when you feel unable to deal with what the day throws at you.

Sleep scientists have become increasingly interested in looking at how these differences in people may affect their health. Whether you are a morning or an evening person is known as your chronotype, and this is relevant to the snooze button. Morning larks have very little sleep inertia and are the most likely to spring out of bed. Night owls will enjoy the snooze button because they do not want to leap out of bed but to stay a while longer. In the 1970s, sleep scientists coined the term 'drockling' to describe this, the gentle drifting in and out of sleep in the early morning. This is exactly what happens when you use your snooze button. You are drockling; the word's ugliness describes fairly well what happens.

The more you drockle, the more confused your body feels: should it prepare for the day or prepare for a night's rest? What you should do is set your alarm for when you need to get up. This may need to include some time to swing your legs over the side of the bed and become fully awake. You should do this every day. Eventually your body should get used to this routine. If you use a snooze button regularly, then you have trained yourself to rely on it, instead of getting up at the first alarm.

## Summary

The snooze button may feel like a good idea but it can also be problematic. Your body is designed to wake up and then be as alert as you need to be in preparation for the day. The snooze confuses your body, your hormones, your energy levels. It tricks your mind into thinking you can achieve another sleep cycle, but the next alarm call in 5 or 10 minutes' time has different ideas.

The resulting effect is about you as an individual. If it works for you then it's hard to see it as a negative effect. However, if it still leaves you feeling you need more sleep then it is probably not working. The key is going to sleep early enough for you to have a natural feeling of being awake at approximately the time you need to get up, though the change to routine this implies may not be good news for everyone.

## Top tips

1 Do you use a snooze button on a regular basis and feel you need those snoozes to prepare you for the shock of getting out of bed? Why not try without? My wife used to love her snooze button to get up for work, at what felt like an unnaturally early wake-up time for her. She invested in a light alarm clock, which has a light that gradually brightens up for 30 minutes before the alarm goes off. The light signals allow the body to wake up gradually with the light, so you are often awake or almost awake before the alarm goes off. All right, it does still have a snooze button, but she now doesn't go back to sleep once the alarm goes off, yet can still enjoy some time in bed thinking about the day without the risk of falling asleep and being late for work!

2 If you feel really bad in the morning getting up with the alarm, you may not be getting enough total sleep. Try bringing your bedtime forward gradually until you reach a point at which you are able to feel awake when your alarm goes off.

# 5

# 'I yawn because I'm tired'

A yawn happens when we involuntarily open our mouths, take a deep inhalation of air, followed by a deep exhalation. In English the name is an onomatopoeia: it sounds like the actual object and you can see yourself yawning when you say the word. During the yawn your eardrums are stretched a little, and sometimes you make other bodily movements, including swallowing. A yawn is a response, an automatic reaction, that we have little control over; once a yawn has started, it is very difficult, or may even be impossible, to stop it.

You are likely to yawn when you see someone else yawn, particularly when you watch his or her eyes, when you hear yawning or when you think about a yawn. You may even yawn when you see your dog or cat yawn; it is that contagious. I am fighting the urge to yawn right now, while I write this chapter, and when I told my family, my sister-in-law started yawning away. I took this to be a contagion rather than a comment on my conversational skills. I bet many of you are yawning as you read these lines (though I do sincerely hope that's not a reflection on the quality of my writing).

Different cultures have different beliefs about what yawning means. A yawn may be culturally inappropriate because it is thought to allow good spirits loose from your open mouth. This superstition may be related to a public-health need for more careful sanitation and behaviours. In British culture, though, yawning is associated with two states: when you are bored or when you feel tired. Let's deal first with the idea that yawning is a sign of boredom. Derren Brown, a very talented illusionist and mentalist (not sure what that means, but that's how his website describes his profession), has produced some breathtaking acts, described in his book *Tricks of the Mind*, published in 2006. He does not worry if people yawn during his shows. As an entertainer he does not consider it a reason to be concerned. He is far more concerned with coughing as a sign of boredom. Anecdotally I can attest to this. When I am in large lecture theatres teaching some complex material that can be boring to student doctors, I note coughing as a reliable sign that I need to change tack. I don't understand how boredom became associated with yawning, and there is no evidence this is real.

## So why do we yawn?

All humans yawn, as do many other animals: cats and dogs yawn, as the thousands of YouTube videos can show you. It must be an important activity but nobody seems totally sure about why we do it. The definition in dictionaries is that it is a response to tiredness or boredom but there is no evidence to support this. There are a fair number of hypotheses as to why we yawn, all of which seem plausible but none of which has been proved.

The first one is that your blood contains the dissolved gas carbon dioxide, and when this rises over a certain threshold, the yawn allows a large influx of oxygen and dumping of carbon dioxide. The flaw with this theory is that when you increase or decrease the levels of oxygen and carbon dioxide, the amount of yawning does not change. You can even test this yourself: hold your breath for a very short while and this will not result in a yawn. If you swim, and dive underwater for a swim, you will have no urge to yawn when you resurface.

A second hypothesis, favoured by anthropologists, stresses the potential cultural and social role of yawning. The contagious yawn has been proposed as a way of keeping a group of humans safe, ready to respond to any danger. The yawn may be a way to remind all members of a group to stay alert, particularly as the day rolls on and tiredness begins to have an impact. This is supported by the fact that members of the parachute infantry waiting to jump from an aircraft tend to yawn more, which may be preparation for feelings of fear and terror.

A third possible reason is that yawning controls the temperature of the brain or even of the whole body. When you put cold packs on people, they yawn less. A fourth, more recent idea comes from observations that yawning may be some complex reaction to chemicals in the body. Various drugs, both prescribed and recreational, seem to induce a yawn, including selective serotonin reuptake inhibitors (SSRIs), used to treat depression and anxiety, but the reason for this is not clear.

A fifth possible reason, from social science, is that the group yawn may simply be a way for the group to demonstrate empathy for each other, maintaining the bond between people. A scientific project found that children with autistic spectrum disorder do not seem to catch the need to yawn in the same way.

## Yawning to clean your tonsils

A really interesting hypothesis, and the one that seems most plausible, suggests that yawning is used to clean the tonsils: the tonsillar evacuation hypothesis. This is because a yawn contracts the muscles in the mouth and particularly the throat, which could then eject debris from the tonsils. We are aware of the sensation as it happens, without the need to do anything. The contraction prevents a build-up of material, which could lead to infections. In fact the yoga exercise Simhasana may be useful to achieve the same benefit, where you stretch your throat muscles to the extreme and it is said to help get rid of a throat infection.

This hypothesis also has an explanation for why we relate yawning to tiredness. The theory suggests that the yawn is an important process, and should happen frequently. However, it is not critical that it happens at a specific point in time, just as long as we do it often enough to keep the tonsils clean. A yawn would be an inconvenient thing to happen when your survival might depend on doing something it would hamper. So it is best to yawn during an inactive period in your day: preparing for bed seems a good time, the time in your body clock when your body is relaxing, when you feel contented and safe, which also coincides with when you feel most sleepy.

## Summary

We do not know with certainty why we yawn, but it is not really an indication of boredom or of tiredness. A plausible reason is that your body yawns when it is most relaxed, often around the same time you prepare for sleep. I like the idea that you are continually cleaning your tonsils by yawning.

## Top tips

1 If you are concerned about people being bored, look out for the coughing, not yawning.
2 Don't feel embarrassed and try to stifle a yawn; relish the fact that you may be cleaning your tonsils and staving off a throat infection!

# 6

# 'I must sleep in one continuous block of time'

As will be described in more detail in Chapter 12, we have changed our sleep patterns dramatically over the past few centuries. There is historical evidence in plays and stories, and in the language used, that our ancestors did not sleep in a single continuous block of time. We have this idea that once your head hits the pillow, you should next wake and then rise from bed after a single continuous block of sleep. This type of continuous sleep is known as monophasic sleep, 'mono' meaning 'one'. Makes it sound very clever, but there is evidence that this may not be biologically the only, or ideal, approach.

This idea that monophasic sleep may not be perfect has intrigued many people over the years. When looking back at our ancestors, the evidence suggests that we took a first sleep, then a break of a significant period of time, followed by the second, also known as dead sleep. The length of time each of these phases lasted is not clear, but a 4-hour first sleep would probably be completely normal, as that fits with the core human sleep. The length of the second sleep was more likely to differ based on location on the Earth and the time of year. The closer you are to the poles, the more change there is in the light–dark cycle. In the UK, for example, we have nights that last up to 18 hours in the middle of winter, and in summer it is just 6 hours.

There is an increasingly active group of people who are changing their sleep habits and patterns, and we will spend a little time describing some of the most extreme activities of this community of special sleepers. On some social media websites, enthusiasts discuss the approaches you can take to managing your time asleep. Indeed, humans must be able to deal with dramatic changes in the environment and the cues they give us that run our body clock, known as zeitgebers (see Chapter 15 for more detail on these cues and how they operate to manage our waking and sleeping life). The significant changes we make to our lives and the timing of events, with work shift patterns, staying up late, jetting around the world, show that we can deal with sleep patterns that diverge considerably from the modern standard.

## Many people try to manipulate their sleep patterns

If you take more than one phase of sleep you are taking what is called polyphasic sleep, which is often seen as a way to become more flexible with time, creating space for more work, more family, more social time. Chapter 30 looks at what the extra time in your day might mean. If you think you can operate on less sleep, the time you save has been equated to having a full-time assistant. There are also claims from some of the enthusiasts that the manipulations may reduce insomnia, but there does not seem to be any scientific backing for this.

Two phases of sleep, similar to what is described in Chapter 12, is known as segmented sleep or biphasic sleep. This type is thought to be the most natural form of sleep. Both periods of sleep are at night-time, during nocturnal hours. It has been suggested that after getting used to this pattern, you may have a change in your energy levels and mental aptitude. People living in Mediterranean countries have historically adopted a two-phase sleep schedule, using a siesta, in which a short sleep of 30–90 minutes is taken after a hearty lunch. Business closes for this time, over the hottest time of the day, and the community settles down for a rest.

## There are many different types of polyphasic sleep

Many people have developed different ways of manipulating their sleep, with various systems based on some evidence, thought and experience. They have given the different systems attractive and appealing names. One of the most popular sleep schedules is known as the Everyman schedule. This pattern attempts to use your daily body rhythm and what are known as ultradian rhythms. Ultradian rhythms are repeating patterns within the day, like the 90 or so minutes of the sleep stages. There are different types of Everyman schedules; for instance, the Everyman 2 has a core sleep of 4.5 to 6 hours in the middle of the night, with two 20-minute naps. Higher-numbered Everyman schedules (3 and 4) consist of a shortened core sleep and three or four naps in the day.

There are other sleep schedules, in which you sleep for more than one period of time during the night. You could try a dual-core sleep, with a short sleep around dusk and one around dawn. Dual-core sleep is supplemented by some naps. This is fairly similar to a biphasic overnight with the addition of a traditional siesta. This simple system aligns a little with your body clock – what is known as the circadian rhythm (see Chapter 15 for more details).

The 'Uberman sleep schedule' became one of the most frequently attempted sleep schedules. Uberman sleep is where there are no core periods of sleep; you do not take any extended sleep during the night. It is based on a series of short naps through the 24 hours. Conventionally this will be between six and eight 20-minute naps. When you add these periods up, it totals around 2–3 hours of total sleep time in the 24 hours, giving a dramatic increase in the amount of time you are not sleeping.

## Downsides and upsides of polyphasic sleep

There are undoubtedly potential downsides of the managed sleep schedules. Critics point to a lack of understanding about how your brain can adapt to a series of shorter periods of sleep, or naps, for the critical roles sleep plays in your daily life. They also propose that your body will revolt and not allow anything but a single sleep phase. Some people who suffer from insomnia may not agree with this. Either way, there hasn't been sufficient research to know which view is correct. To some extent this comes back to a fundamental unknown, namely that we do not completely understand why we sleep, so cannot know whether or not manipulating sleep can cause harm.

One possible upside lies in the way your productivity might be enhanced; that is, how much work you can get done. You may not choose to manipulate your sleep for that reason, but if you were to, some people think that, after a nap, you can work well for another few hours, and that this may also increase creativity. This all boils down to how much work you want to do, and how important working is to you.

Some thought must be given to the timing of your core sleep within one of these schedules. The stages of sleep are discussed more fully in Chapter 20, but it is clear that the critical stage of deep sleep is less likely to take place from 3 a.m. to 8 a.m. in the early morning.

## Summary

Most people sleep in a single continuous period, but there are many other options that change the amount you sleep and when. The different schedules use what we know about the body clock. There are some potential positive reasons for using a polyphasic sleep schedule, often revolving around the extra time they free up during the day, but there are downsides – in particular, the fact that we do not know what the long-term effects of these sleep patterns may be.

## Top tips

1 Think about your sleep pattern using a sleep diary (see Chapter 1). Do you have a single- or two-phase sleep schedule naturally? If you do wake in the night, don't feel this is abnormal. It may be an entirely rational way to sleep. Indeed it may be more natural than one sleep.
2 Be wary of trying alternative polyphasic sleep patterns. Think about what you are trying to achieve by doing this and if that is necessary. Bear in mind that we do not know what effects this will have in the long term.

# 7

# 'I tried mindfulness once and it didn't help me to sleep'

How often have you got into bed ready to sleep and suddenly remembered something you forgot to do that day? Before you know it, your mind has magnified the thing. You are suddenly thinking about all the consequences of your error; the last thing your mind wants to do is go to sleep. No doubt you can think of several times this has happened. Using logic, it is easy to see that any error is in the past, any consequences are in the future and there is probably nothing you can do right at that moment to alter these facts, but how often are we rational in these situations? This is where practising mindfulness can be helpful.

If you have ever wondered what mindfulness entails, it is an activity conducted in your mind that is designed to help you deal with your life. You may have seen advertising where you live, marketing local sessions in mindfulness and meditation. It is an expanding industry, even including a growing one in colouring books described as being mindful.

When we think of meditation, we often imagine a Buddhist monk, draped in saffron robes, sitting in quiet contemplation on a mountain top. Mindfulness, which is a form of meditation, is about knowing what is happening here and now, when it is happening, no matter what is happening; this is the practical definition of mindfulness meditation.

Mindfulness is not about emptying your mind. It is the opposite of being mindless or on automatic pilot. It is about having your mind full, full of the present experience. When you are present, you allow yourself to stop thinking, to quieten your mind from the constant chatter, to focus on the now.

It requires practice, and you will need to expend some effort. I know that the first few sessions I did had little noticeable impact. In fact I had to fight the urge to fall asleep, which is not the intention. You might be questioning at this point why I have included mindfulness in a book about how to sleep better and then said that the aim of mindfulness is not to fall asleep. As will be explained, mindfulness is a conscious process of being during your waking hours, which with practice will lead to a calmer mind. Once you have achieved this, your sleep will naturally improve.

## What is mindfulness-based therapy?

Mindfulness practice involves paying attention to the moment you are experiencing. The way you pay attention is more important than what you see. Try to pay attention to all your different senses: the sounds you hear, what you see, how your body feels physically, what emotions you are feeling. Just stop right now and take notice of everything around you: the sights, sounds, smells and so on. You might become aware of the fact that we rarely do this; we are often so caught up in our thoughts that we fail to notice what is going on around us at any given moment.

Shane uses mindfulness-based therapy in his work, as it is an effective treatment for a variety of psychological issues. In his clinic he asks people 'How do you feel?' 'Fine!' they often reply. This is an answer that is often the opposite of what a person is feeling. Once you move to a more honest description of the feelings you are experiencing, he can ask not only 'How do you feel?' but also 'How do you feel about how you feel?'

When you are worried about a meeting the following day, do you feel as though you need to worry? This uncovers the idea that worry gives the illusion you are doing something about an issue when actually you are not. The worry takes you away from the present moment.

Feelings can overwhelm you at times, but with mindfulness you can see yourself as more than just a collection of thoughts, experiences and feelings. When your attention is focused, you are not slipping back into the past and how things could have been different. When you are mindful, your focus stays in the present and is not concerned with the creation of an alternative past, present or future. These 'If only . . . then . . .' statements are disarmed by mindfulness.

## First practise mindfulness with your bedtime routine

There are many ways to develop your skills in being mindful. An excellent starting point is to make it part of your everyday activities. How about, the next time you prepare for bed, which is usually a mindless experience, trying to do it mindfully? As you pick up your pyjamas, how do they feel? What is the temperature of the room like? How bright are the lights? As you climb into bed, what noise does this make? What is the colour, the texture of the pillow?

As you then start to sink into your bed, try to be engulfed by the experience; focus on the warmth, the feelings of heaviness you have. Think only about that experience; do not give thought to anything else. When a thought comes into your mind (and it will), label it as a 'thought', allow it to have its space, and bring your attention back to the activity of getting into bed. You will notice that the thought drifts away.

One aspect of mindfulness that is critical to sleep is taking a non-judgemental stance. Think about only the present moment, just the facts. Don't judge these – for example, don't think about why it was so rainy today when yesterday was warm and sunny, or wonder what is making a particular noise. Try to accept things for what they are. The goal is to help manage how our experiences, such as the mood we are in, or our opinions can influence the present moment.

## Summary

There is evidence that mindfulness meditation can work. It is true that a single session will not have an immediate impact; it is a practice that requires time and effort. This chapter has offered a brief introduction to mindfulness and how being mindful can influence your mood and help your sleep. Practising these techniques can help, moving you from being mindless and on automatic pilot to being present and full of the current experience.

## Top tips

1 Take part in learning mindfulness meditation. There are some excellent books, courses and YouTube videos you could try;

some are listed at the end of the book. This needs work, and you have to commit the time.

2 Try being mindful when you wake in the night and want to return to sleep. Focus on your breath; feel the cool air; feel the movement across your nose. Be engulfed by the activity; if a thought enters your mind, allow it to just be; don't tease it apart.

# 8

# 'Your head can explode while you sleep'

There is a condition known as exploding head syndrome. This does sound terrible and, thank goodness, is not a precise description, but it is a name for a real condition with traumatic symptoms that can cause distress to those who suffer from it. The syndrome is characterized by the person hearing a very loud noise, often happening just before he or she falls asleep or when waking during the night. This noise can sound like an explosion or gunfire, so the description represents the feeling that those who have it experience from this condition.

You may have experienced being woken by a loud noise. I certainly have. Of course, it is dark and everyone else in the house is asleep, which means I cannot check with someone if the sound was real, but I think that I sometimes experience a mild version of the syndrome.

Exploding head syndrome is what is known as a parasomnia, which is a disorder of sleep in which your nervous system does not act as it should. This is the same as for sleepwalking (see Chapter 11). Looking at the world we now live in, we might expect the name to have a relatively modern origin, but the syndrome was first described in 1876 and the term was coined in 1920. The name represents how loud and disturbing this noise can be – it can feel like an explosion going off in your head. The syndrome is rare and has been reported in people of any age. A quarter of young adults interviewed said they had experienced it at least once, however. It does also seem to be more prevalent in women.

Thankfully these episodes are usually brief, although they can cause distress and anxiety. Science has not discovered why they happen or the mechanism involved, but, rest assured, your head does not explode.

## Summary

Your head won't blow up; the name is a rather visual description of a horrid and thankfully rare condition.

## Top tip

1  You should not worry about hearing weird and unexpected sounds during the night. Many people hear sounds at night; you are not unusual.

# 9

# 'Holding a spoon allows me to nap'

I was telling one of my PhD students about this book you are now reading and she replied: 'Oh, you must have heard about the spoon and the nap.' I immediately thought she was talking about what is known as the multiple sleep onset latency test. This was invented by the pioneer of sleep research, Dr William C. Dement, when trying to develop objective measurements of all things sleep. He wanted a simple measure of how long after lying down and closing your eyes it takes you to fall asleep.

This is not as straightforward as you might think. Defining the time you close your eyes is easy, not difficult to work out, but what about the time you fall asleep? This is not an easily defined point. Dement came up with a simple method – there are more details of this in Chapter 3.

Anyway, it turns out my student was not talking about a scientific method but an actual method that people use to manage their sleep. This is known as the drop nap.

It operates in a similar way to the objective sleep measure. The sleeper holds a spoon over a plate, but rather than measuring something, chooses to wake when the spoon drops from the hand. When the spoon strikes the plate, making a loud noise, the sleeper wakes up and continues with his or her day.

It is a simple alarm clock that is tied in to your physiological state. This whole concept sounds odd, but perhaps if you plan to take a nap, you should keep it relatively short and avoid straying into the deep stage of sleep (see Chapter 20 for a more detailed look at sleep stages). In the deep-sleep stage your muscles relax and at that point the spoon should fall. That's a guess, but it is probably the intention. Your muscles relax before you enter the deep-sleep stage, and probably before sleep itself.

## Summary

There's nowt so queer as folk.

## Top tips

1 You should probably not regularly nap holding a spoon.
2 Napping may be helpful, so if you feel you can adopt it, see Chapter 19 for a more detailed look at the possible benefits and drawbacks.

# 10

# 'Coffee doesn't affect my sleep'

I like coffee because it gives me the illusion that I might be awake.

Lewis Black

Cappuccino, flat white, piccolo, long black, latte, Americano – whatever your favourite, we can probably all agree that there has been an explosion in the 'coffee culture' across the world. From Australians, who decided to be clear and descriptive with the flatness and length of their drinks, to the Italians, who sneer at anything but espresso after lunchtime, we are obsessed with this drink.

According to the European Coffee Federation, 725 million cups of coffee are consumed in Europe every day, which amounts to 4 kilograms (a little under 9 pounds) of coffee per person per year. Most adults in westernized societies eat and drink it on a frequent basis. For example, 90 per cent of Americans are thought to consume caffeine every day. By 2020 there are predicted to be 21,000 coffee shops in the UK.

Coffee and tea drinking have been around for a long time. The earliest evidence of humans drinking coffee is in the fifteenth century, in Yemen in the Middle East, where coffee beans were exported from their place of origin in Ethiopia in Africa. The pastime of coffee drinking reached Persia and Turkey in the sixteenth century, moving to the rich in Venice in Italy and then the rest of Europe. The word 'coffee' was probably from an Arabic word *qahwah*. Soon after this, coffee houses opened across much of urban Europe, then spreading across the world. Balliol College in Oxford claim that one of their former students, Nathanael Konopios, introduced coffee to the UK in the early seventeenth century.

## Coffee has physical effects on us

As you probably know, coffee contains the drug caffeine, which is the most widely consumed mind-affecting – or psycho-active –

drug in the world. Caffeine occurs naturally in many plants, not just the coffee bean. In fact, over 60 plant species contain caffeine, including tea and cocoa, used to make chocolate. Tea seems to have been around for longer than coffee. Legend has it that a Chinese emperor noted that when tea leaves fell into boiling water it produced a pleasant fragrance, starting the world's love of tea.

Caffeine is a stimulant. It increases blood pressure and prevents or slows down drowsiness, producing increased alertness and focus. We think this is a fun drug: it is legal; fairly cheap; does useful things. According to the 2001 Sleep in America poll, 43 per cent of Americans are 'very likely' to use caffeinated beverages to combat daytime sleepiness. These are the main reasons we drink coffee over and above just a pleasant taste.

Once you swallow food or drink, it passes into the stomach and your body immediately tries to digest and absorb all it can. Absorbed caffeine then moves into your blood, and it can begin its work on your mind after 15 minutes. This speed is also a reason why some over-the-counter pain relief medicines have caffeine added.

All drugs have what is called a half-life. It is the time it takes for half of the drug to be removed from the bloodstream by the organs in your body, such as the liver. For caffeine, this is around 6 hours. That means that many, many hours after drinking your coffee or eating that piece of chocolate, there is still some caffeine coursing through your veins and arteries.

As well as making you feel more alert, you may also notice your heart beating more quickly; you may also need to wee more often. When the caffeine reaches your brain, it increases norepinephrine, which is a hormone that controls panic. These effects can be useful when you need to react with urgency, but have less use in your normal day-to-day activity.

## Are there any adverse health effects?

As a society, we underestimate the power of caffeine and its associated impacts. As a reflective society, we are concerned that the liquids we consume may cause cancer or have some other harmful effects on our health.

In 1991, the World Health Organization's International Agency for Research on Cancer, the organization in charge of checking whether or not chemicals cause cancer, said there was no evidence that caffeine caused cancer. It did report, however, after reviewing very limited evidence, that coffee was a possible carcinogen to the bladder. Don't be alarmed by this, though, as by 2010, over 500 studies on cancer and coffee had been published. These found that coffee might, in fact, reduce the risks of some cancers, including endometrial, and even reduce your risk of liver cancer by 50 per cent. So, some positive news, but it is still good for us to moderate our intake.

There has been some concern about drinking coffee during pregnancy particularly, as it seems that many pregnant women are naturally unable to contemplate drinking any coffee because of nausea. Good scientific evidence shows that moderate consumption, classified as no more than two standard cups per day, is not harmful to the growing foetus. The American College of Obstetricians and Gynecologists advise that less than 200 milligrams of caffeine per day, or one standard cup from your favourite café, causes no harm to the baby.

You must also be mindful of how many other drinks contain caffeine. Tea, cola and energy drinks, under their many different brand names, all contain caffeine. The amount of caffeine varies depending on how much you drink and how you make the drink. Tea has roughly half of the caffeine content of a filter coffee, but more than an average can of cola.

Coffee manufacturers were aware of the effect of caffeine, therefore the process of removing caffeine from coffee to make decaffeinated coffee was invented at the start of the twentieth century. Tea manufacturers then produced caffeine-free tea, given the demand for it from the public.

I realized many years ago that I was getting a splitting headache only on Saturdays. I put this down to all sorts of causes, such as the sports I played at the weekend or the hangover from the night before, but I have now realized, after not playing sport and not getting drunk, that it must be something else. I do drink lots of coffee on weekdays, either at work or in the local cafés. At the weekend I spend more time with the family. On top of this, we drink decaffeinated coffee at home. These things mean that my body has withdrawal symptoms from my weekday caffeine habit at the weekend.

## Sleep disorders may be related to caffeine

It is amazing how many people think that caffeine has no effect on their sleep. It is a common cause of difficulties, yet there would be a huge impact on society if coffee was banned. I enjoy a coffee as much as the next person, but the evidence suggests that consuming caffeine is a bad approach to sleep management and there are some ways in which we can improve the situation.

The effect of caffeine on sleep seems to vary hugely between people. Some people can drink a double espresso immediately before bed and then sleep, whereas others who have only one cup of coffee in the day find their sleep affected. For some people, drinking too much coffee is thought to cause a type of intoxication – the person is unable to rest, remain calm, think clearly or speak without rambling.

People who consume excessive amounts of caffeine, particularly before bedtime, may suffer from a psychiatric disorder known as caffeine-induced sleep disorder. The onset of sleep, once you have taken to your bed, may be delayed, which is known as sleep-onset latency.

The stages of sleep that we have been able to identify in the laboratory may be altered. Rapid eye movement (REM) sleep, which is thought to be related to dreaming, may be reduced. Perhaps more worryingly, the deep sleep, which is called slow-wave sleep by sleep scientists, seems to be reduced in the hours after drinking coffee. Reduced slow-wave sleep has impacts on learning, metabolism and heart disease.

A research article published in the *Journal of Clinical Sleep Medicine* found that when caffeine is taken as long as 6 hours before bedtime, it adversely affects sleep. One coffee in the afternoon could stop you from going to sleep normally. Also, it can significantly increase the time taken to fall asleep. The participants slept for 40 minutes less if they had caffeine. Another study found that caffeine does not help alertness after three nights of poor sleep.

## Drinking coffee in modern society

Doctors think that children should not consume caffeine (although, having raised children, I hope that referred to coffee and not chocolate). Coffee has no real nutrient benefit and not introducing the drink should have no impact.

Is there perhaps a real positive to people frequenting cafés as opposed to pubs or bars? Coffee houses are starting to replace the alcohol-drinking culture, certainly in the UK. The key is that people socialize in a safe environment with friends, providing warmth, relaxation, togetherness. Any business needs to make money to survive and so it makes sense that they are selling something. In this case, they are selling coffee, often with posh types of tea and chocolate and cake.

Are caffeine-based drinks safer than alcohol-based ones? There is clear evidence that they are, when compared to the appalling effects of alcoholism and its damage to internal organs such as the liver and heart. This is in addition to related incidence of violence, drink-driving, antisocial behaviour and abuse.

## Summary

All the evidence suggests that caffeine does have physiological effects on the body, but whether this translates into difficulties getting off to sleep or not seems to vary from person to person. The study described shows that caffeine does affect sleep when measured in a lab, and it may be that it has effects on everyone's sleep, but some people are able to tolerate this without feeling 'wired'. It is reassuring to know that there don't seem to be any serious long-term effects from drinking coffee, although children and pregnant women should be careful and restrict their consumption.

## Top tips

1 You have seen that caffeine affects sleep. Why don't you try cutting out caffeine as far as you can from your diet? Try cutting out coffee and tea – drink decaffeinated instead – for 2 weeks, then try the sleep diary again to see if the time you spend asleep improves and if there is a difference to how you feel in the day. My wife used to believe that coffee didn't affect her; she never got 'that buzz' from drinking a cup. However, when she cut out caffeine completely, her sleep improved dramatically. Give it a go. The results may surprise you!

2 Don't forget that caffeine isn't only found in tea and coffee. Cola drinks and chocolate both contain caffeine, as do other things you may not expect.

3 Try to stop drinking caffeine by 3 p.m., if your normal bedtime is between 9 p.m. and midnight.

# 11

## 'Don't wake a sleepwalker'

GENTLEWOMAN   I have seen her rise from her bed, throw her night-
gown upon her . . . yet all this while in a most fast
sleep [. . .]
DOCTOR   You see her eyes are open.
GENTLEWOMAN   Ay, but their sense is shut.

William Shakespeare, *Macbeth*, Act V, Scene 1

Sleepwalking, known in clinical circles as somnambulism or noc-
tambulism, is fascinating and scary in equal measure. Knowledge
of this led William Shakespeare to set Lady Macbeth sleepwalking
in her final scene on stage.

When sleepwalking, you are asleep, your brain is asleep but,
usually, your eyes are open. Your gaze is different from your normal
waking, focused attention. You may look towards someone, but
this is described as staring straight through him or her, with no
acknowledgement, no recognition. There are many anecdotes of
the range of activities and behaviours, ranging from mundane
to bizarre. You may perform simple tasks, repetitive tasks or
sometimes quite complex activities – even driving a car has been
reported.

An episode may last only a few minutes or much longer. After
sleepwalking, people may wake in a bath (like one of my daughters), having refolded their sheets and clothes (like a friend), in
hospital as a result of having fallen over (again a friend) or find they
have left the house (which a patient did). Because it is out of the
ordinary, there are sceptics – those who think we didn't land on the
Moon and that Elvis is still alive. Nevertheless, when you chat with
people who do sleepwalk, it is anything but pretend. It can feel
disturbing, even terrifying. The feelings stem from failing to recall
the things you did, but having the evidence that you did do them.

If you sleepwalk, it is most likely that your brain is coming around
from the deep-sleep stage (see Chapter 20 for more details of sleep

stages), but your body is not experiencing any paralysis. Paralysis, which is entirely normal, stops you from moving too much while you sleep and may happen during the rapid eye movement (REM) stage of your sleep to stop you acting out your dreams.

## Sleepwalking usually starts at a young age

Young people are the most likely to sleepwalk. Reports estimate that around a fifth of children will sleepwalk at least once. Usually most people grow out of this by the time they reach puberty, but not everyone does. Sleepwalking can continue for the rest of their lives, which is when it can become a serious issue.

Apart from youngsters being particularly vulnerable, we don't know much about the causes. It does run in families, but often people who sleepwalk have no family members who exhibit the behaviour. Sleepwalking has some triggers, such as being overtired, stressed or anxious. Some infections, imbibing too much alcohol and some drugs, both legal and illegal, may cause an episode.

## What to do with a sleepwalker

The most critical part of dealing with a sleepwalker is to make sure the person is safe. People sleepwalking are mobile, moving around rooms, using stairs or sitting down doing some activity. You can gently wake them if there is a hazard, but gradually guiding them back to their bed will often be sufficient. Also, a good idea may be – when they have stopped their sleepwalking and are back in a safe place – gently to wake them fully. This is the best way to prevent the same sleep cycle returning them to a further bout of walking.

## Summary

Sleepwalking is real; it is not a convenient dramatic tool. It is also not unusual – a large proportion of people report at least one sleep-walk in their life. Gently returning them to their room is the best approach. Waking them is not dangerous, but they may feel dis-orientated and confused.

## Top tip

There is no tip in this chapter for sleeping better. If you are a sleep-walker, then please see your general practitioner if you have not done so already. Stay safe.

# 12

# 'I haven't slept well if I woke during the night'

You have work in the morning and have set your alarm for the usual time. You don't have much trouble falling asleep but before you know it, you have woken up. You glance at your clock only to discover it is some god-awful time in the early hours. A quick calculation and you work out you have slept for 4 hours. That is not enough!

What are you going to do? If you lie still, surely you will fall comfortably back to sleep? Before you know it, you are thinking about that difficult meeting at work; and the trouble you are having with your friend; and the nightmare neighbour. Your mind is on fire. Your body wants to move and your mind is racing; the last thing you can do is fall back to sleep.

Sound familiar?

This pattern of waking has different names, such as 'middle-of-the-night insomnia', 'wake-after-sleep-onset' or sometimes 'sleep maintenance insomnia'. We define this in various ways, but most commonly it is when someone wakes after having had some sleep. The time awake varies but the accepted definition is that you are awake for at least 30 minutes during the night. You might awaken after a short sleep, of say 30–60 minutes, or more commonly after around 3–4 hours.

## Middle-of-the-night insomnia is common

If I were a betting man I would lay money on the fact that you know someone who has described this to you, or maybe it has happened to you. Middle-of-the-night insomnia is one of the more frequent sleep complaints I hear. This is not just anecdotally true; surveys suggest this is the most common sleep complaint, too.

Labelling broken sleep 'insomnia' implies that it is problematic.

The public believes a long stretch of unbroken sleep is a birthright, and that any break in sleep needs to be addressed. Unfortunately, many doctors also assume the same.

A US study of over 8,000 adults published in 2008 found that 35 per cent of people woke during the night at least three times per week. Waking during the night is not just an American phenomenon: an extensive UK online survey from 2012 reported that 32 per cent described waking at night. These awakenings seem to be more prevalent in women and are possibly more common in older people than in the young.

What causes us to wake? Some people have underlying health issues, such as pain from arthritis or restless legs syndrome. Pregnancy can also be related to more frequent night waking. You will wake up if you need to use the toilet, but this does not automatically lead to remaining awake. Most people who experience waking in the night do not have these underlying issues.

It may lead to difficulties the following day: tiredness and lethargy; impaired ability to complete activities. It may also lead to your taking more daytime naps: over 20 per cent of the general public report that they nap at least a few days per week. These issues also inevitably lead to more sick leave.

## We may always have slept in two stages

It is fair to say that we assume sleep should happen in a single, unbroken period at night, but that has not always been the case. In fact it was not the standard pattern until very recently. The expert thinking is that, until the last two centuries, we used to have our sleep broken naturally in the middle of the night. The first part of the sleep, known imaginatively as 'first sleep', may have been around 4 hours in length. It seems that there was then a period of being awake, perhaps around 1–2 hours, when people would have been fairly active. They may have chatted with bedfellows, had sex, offered prayers to their gods, even got up to move around. There are late fifteenth-century prayers written specifically for use in the hours in between the two sleep periods. The time and activity following the first sleep was sometimes referred to as the 'watch'.

This was then followed by a second sleep, which would run until dawn. In medieval England this was called dead sleep or morning sleep. In modern terminology, such a broken sleep pattern is known as segmented sleep or biphasic sleep pattern. This sounds a little like the description in *The Lord of the Rings* of first breakfast and second breakfast, but there is considerable evidence that it was normal. There is even an old English word for the gentle slumber we enjoy in the morning: 'sloom'. There are plenty of documents that support this, and a great deal of research was published by the historian Roger Ekirch in 2001. To take an example from literature written many centuries ago: 'Don Quixote followed nature, and being satisfied with his first sleep, did not solicit more. As for Sancho, he never wanted a second, for the first lasted him from night to morning' (Miguel Cervantes, *Don Quixote*, 1615).

The first and second periods of sleep were not just an English activity. There are words in French: *premier somme* describes first sleep; the time between sleep was called *dorveille*, which is a combination of *dormir*, 'to sleep', and *veiller*, 'to be awake'. There are similar phrases in Italian and Latin.

Of course, there was far less artificial lighting available to people before the invention of gas and then electric lighting. Most people would retire to bed around dark and get up shortly before dawn. During the seventeenth century, sleeping habits started to change. With the social changes brought about by the invention of lighting, late-night coffee houses and the well-off being able to use the night-time hours for social activities, there was a complete change in the attitudes towards darkness being a dangerous time. There was no turning back once towns and cities started to light the streets at night. Paris was the first, in 1667, and very swiftly many cities in Europe and further afield invested in this, leading to changes in sleep patterns.

## Summary

The evidence presented here clearly shows that it is a myth that you can't have slept well if you woke in the middle of the night. It seems that historically this was a natural part of life and continues to be the case for many people. The reality is that modern life has interfered with our actual 'normal' sleep, and historical documents suggest that we slept in at least two phases. When you work out how you sleep, as described in Chapter 1, you can then consider your sleep pattern to be completely normal for you. This will allow you to listen to your own body and sleep in a pattern that is right for you.

## Top tips

1  If you are someone who wakes in the night, it would be useful to revisit the sleep diary described in Chapter 1. In addition to recording what time you went to bed and what time you woke in the morning, you should also document what time and for how long you woke during the night. You may find after doing this for a couple of weeks that there is a clear pattern and that you are someone who has a biphasic sleep pattern. If you can then accept that as being right for you, it is no longer a issue that you have to battle against. Work out what is best for you to do during the awake period – reading a book, getting up and doing something or just lying enjoying some solitude.
2  Don't get distressed if you wake in the middle of the night. If anxious or distressing thoughts are waking you, this may need some psychological help (see Chapter 29). If you are just wakeful, accept it for what it is and you will sleep again when you feel tired. The worst thing is to count the hours, getting more and more worried about the lack of time until you need to get up. Enjoy this time.

# 13

# 'My television helps me to sleep'

What hath night to do with sleep?

John Milton, *Comus*

A good question there from John Milton: what has night-time got to do with sleep? Many people tell me that they have their television on at night to help them fall asleep. I remember in the 1980s how my sister was well ahead in the technology stakes by buying a television for her bedroom. A massive clunking behemoth, with dust gathering all over the cathode-ray tube.

So what is the problem? The television provides some company, a device that can push entertainment passively into your mind. The difficulty with it is that it feeds into a fundamental way in which humans operate. We use the environment to give us cues, and these allow the metabolism to know where we are and where we should be. The television gives out light, which makes the body think it must be daytime. Up until recently, we have not had this sort of stimulus. For most of the time humans have existed, we have had the sun, the moon and, more recently, fire.

## Blue light can disrupt your body clock

The light shining into your bedroom contains different wavelengths, which we discern as colour. A significant amount of light that your body recognizes as white light is mostly blue in colour. This 'blue light' is becoming recognized as a major contribution to the body's understanding of what time of day or night it is. The light is detected partly by the cells in your eyes that you look with, but also a set of cells known as photosensitive ganglion cells. These are especially sensitive to blue light. When your eyes detect blue light, they suppress the production of melatonin.

Melatonin, an important chemical you produce for bringing on sleepiness and maintaining your body asleep, is produced during darkness. Light immediately stops your body producing melatonin, and it rapidly disappears from your bloodstream. All devices that give off light are producing some blue light. These include all smartphones and eBook readers. In addition to the light from these devices, there are also hidden effects of sound on the brain. Apart from the obvious issue that sound may keep you awake, there are more subtle effects. You may choose to maintain the volume quite low, but, regardless of this, the sound can stop you from achieving a restful sleep.

In experiments I am conducting, and others are also working on, there is an apparent issue with sound. Even gentle, relatively quiet sounds can lead to stopping deep sleep. It is a relatively complex effect, which relies on sound stimulation during a particular point in the sleep cycle.

## Street lighting and LED lights may affect your sleep

You may have seen a movement towards more ecologically friendly lighting – away from the old bulbs, with a filament that got hot, to a cool LED system. There have been government moves to replace the energy-guzzling incandescent bulb with the LED type. I like the light they give; we use them at home and they last much longer than the old sort.

It seems, however, that every silver lining must have a cloud. The American Medical Association recently put out a statement asking for more care when designing the use of LED lights for on-street lighting. The LED light seems to produce a lot more blue light than the more old-fashioned yellow sodium street lights. The yellow light did not interfere with the hormone production in the same way as LED lighting.

We seem to be most susceptible to the light that LED lights create and it has been estimated to be five times as disruptive to our body clocks as the old sodium lamps. Unfortunately, the street lights outside your house are not usually under your control, but you may also be replacing your home lights with LED ones. Perhaps consider how you might deal with this. Try not to have your room very brightly lit in the evening, and think about lighting that is softer, less white. See if you can turn the strength of the light down in your home.

## Summary

It is common for people to have a television in their bedrooms. The light this produces may affect your body clock, which uses the outside environment to keep you on track. Your eyes are very clever; they pass information to your brain so it knows when to relax for bedtime. The lights from a television, other devices and increasingly the LED lighting in your home and on the street, make it more important than ever to think about your environment.

## Top tips

1 Watch television in a room that is not your bedroom. Do not use your television to get to sleep.
2 Consider the lighting in your home; think about using dimmer switches or lamps in the evening.

# 14

# 'If dolphins slept, they wouldn't be able to breathe'

'What has this to do with my sleep?' you may ask. Well, nothing; but it's interesting. Some people told me that dolphins don't sleep and Terry Pratchett once wrote that we should not trust them as they grin all the time. I was intrigued, and thought I should look into this, especially as I am now beginning to lose my trust in these wondrous creatures.

Dolphins, like whales and humans, are mammals. They must breathe air into their lungs. Imagine what it would be like if you had to hold your breath until it was 'safe' to breathe. This uncertainty is part of a dolphin's life. Unlike you, they must consciously breathe to make sure they don't take a lungful of seawater. This also means that they cannot go into a full sleep, in which they would not be conscious of what was going on around them. If you tried to sleep in open water, you would quickly drown, or not sleep. Either would lead rapidly to your death.

When you sleep you do not consciously breathe; you are surrounded by air, not water. Your body breathes in and out without a care. This circumstance is not the same for dolphins. Scientists were intrigued, especially since sleep is so important for other mammals, such as yourself. When researchers watched dolphins, they observed them having a resting state either moving little or swimming in a slow circle, over and over again. The blowhole remains above the level of the water, gently blowing out and breathing in. In shallow water they may rest on the seabed, rising now and then to breathe, but this doesn't tell us how they remain able to breathe.

## Scientists discovered the secret

One of the amazing aspects of my job is that I can make discoveries, breakthroughs no human has made before. A breakthrough occurred when scientists attached sensors to a dolphin. They discovered dolphins do an amazing thing: they sleep on just one side; one half of their brain is asleep. The sleeping side of the brain shuts down and has a pattern of brain activity that we associate with sleep. The other half stays active and allows the animal to breathe consciously. This deactivation also allows slow-wave sleep or deep sleep, the same as you or I experience.

The dolphins' environment is so hostile to air-breathing mammals that they only do this for a few minutes, then wake. Later, when the sleep pressure builds and they want to have another rest, the other half of the brain shuts down for a sleep. The pattern repeats throughout the 24 hours of a day, alternating shutting half the brain down, left then right then left. Amazingly they seem to achieve roughly 8 hours' sleep per day, despite the challenging environment.

This weird behaviour – at least, it seems peculiar to us – is even more amazing when you realize that they also close one eye for sleep, and leave one eye open, scanning for danger. The eye on the left closes when they are sleeping on their right-hand side of the brain and vice versa.

Recently it has also been found that some birds sleep while they are flying. Scientists fitted a sensor that measures electrical activity to a bird that flies non-stop, without landing, for 2 months. Like dolphins, they seem to sleep for only seconds and in one half of the brain only.

## Summary

Dolphins perform an amazing feat: they shut down one half, one hemisphere of their brain and sleep in that half only. The other half carries on as normal, scanning for danger and, most importantly, breathing out and in above the water line. Despite their environment, they seem to sleep for around 8 hours.

## Top tips

There is no tip this time – you are not a dolphin; but you could impress a friend with your new-found knowledge.

# 15

## 'Routines are for babies'

When my wife and I were having children, there was some debate and discussion in the media about routine. I don't mean the parents' routine, although I'm sure many improvements could be made there. No, this was about the baby's routine. A line of thinking goes that strict timetables, for feeding, bath and bedtime, work to create a beautiful nirvana of child-rearing. We tried this and it didn't work, not for us.

What about you as an adult? Would a routine help? Let's look at some of the science. Your body has a clock, commonly known as the body clock. It is sometimes used to acknowledge the passage of time, the way you are ageing. This measurement may be more appropriately called a body calendar, with time ticking in hours, days, months and years. You do actually have an inbuilt body clock, known scientifically as the circadian rhythm, or as a biorhythm.

This rhythm is an incredibly important part of your life. As humans we acknowledge its existence, but science is only just beginning to understand its role, let alone how it works. It is not just restricted to humans, nor, in fact, just to animals: plants have time rhythms, too. Perhaps you have seen flowers unfurling in the daylight and receding during darkness. This change is a part of a daily cycle.

### Each cell has a clock

Your body knows where it is, what it should be doing, which hormones are to be pumped into your bloodstream, which should be suppressed. To do this there is a complex method, created by your genes, that counts time. These are known, imaginatively, as clock genes. This clock ticks around to the start again over something like a 25-hour period. The clock follows the daily light-and-dark cycle, a cycle that was so important for our survival historically.

You will be aware of this in simple ways, such as a feeling of tiredness as the evening wears on. Your use of the toilet also changes dramatically overnight – another practical application of your body clock. The clock that we use must be reset as your environment changes through a year. Indeed the whole of long-distance air travel relies on your body being able to reset itself, in the same way that you reset your clocks hanging on a wall.

To do this you use cues, environmental triggers, to make it clear to your body where you are in the day or night. In fact much of the advice on how to manage your time in relation to your sleep pattern is based on managing these cues. They are known as zeitgebers; this is German for 'time giver'.

Zeitgebers are used by your body to manage your body clock, a process known as entrainment. The most obvious zeitgebers are the light-and-dark cycle. You are very aware of this, as it makes you feel awake or tired. Other more subtle cues include temperature, which is why with babies and adults alike we are advised to keep a cool bedroom.

There are loads of other cues, such as the frequency with which you eat food. This is one reason why breaking your fast in the morning is a biologically important process. Social interactions, and exercise, keep your body understanding where you are in your 24-hour day. Your body may use many other cues, such as settling to watch television in the evening or sitting on your daily commute to work. All these keep your body in line with the day and night.

## What can interfere with your routine

A host of factors can interfere with your body clock. You may have experienced jet lag, when you cross timelines around the globe. Your body is quite clear where it thinks it should be, but the actual time has changed. The confusion comes about when zeitgebers are not even close to where your body was expecting them.

You won't experience jet lag that often, unless you work as a pilot or air steward, but confusion also happens when you work shifts. Your body might be expecting a slowing of pace and a bed, but your job demands alertness and complete attention. This is where your body clock becomes confused. So setting up a routine could be important to help you manage your sleep and waking.

Shift work is a major issue for modern society. We absolutely rely on 24-hour electricity, water, the internet, healthcare, aeroplanes and police to name but a few. Business sees profit in longer and longer opening hours, for manufacturing, deliveries, service, food and drink and retail. More and more people are working hours that do not precisely coincide with their circadian rhythm. This is an increasingly important public health issue as the consequences for our health become apparent.

## Summary

You have a body clock, governed by your genes, that works out how to keep you on track with the time of day or night. It uses environmental cues known as zeitgebers to keep your body finely tuned to the day. This can go wrong with extreme, rarer events – jet lag, for example – but other things can interfere, too, such as working shifts.

## Top tips

1 Try to do things in a regular way. Eat food at the same time each day.
2 Set your alarm to wake you at the same time each day. Try even to maintain this over the weekend or when you are not working.

# 16

# 'The more I sleep, the more I need to sleep'

I have heard this myth from many of my medical students. When I delved a little deeper, I found that it stemmed from the case of someone who started sleeping more than they would usually, which then led to the need for even more sleep. The logical extension of this process is an ever-increasing spiral until you can only sleep.

There is no medical or physiological reason for this happening. It may be put down to how we are all different – some of us sleep for 7 hours, others for 9 hours. The 'normal' amount of sleep varies comfortably between 6 and up to 10 hours. To sleep outside of these increases the likelihood of a sleep disorder or some other serious health issue. When you sleep well, whatever the actual amount is, you are comfortable with it, but some people may think that 9 hours is too much, especially if they listen to other people or read articles in the media. It brings us back to the 8-hour sleep myth (see Chapter 1). You don't need 8 hours; you need what you need. Sometimes people may be able to spend less time asleep than they feel comfortable with, but a sleep debt builds and eventually they are forced to return to their natural level.

## There are medical and social reasons for sleeping too much

You might guess that we have a name for sleeping a lot: it is hyper-somnia – though this is when the feelings of tiredness are not relieved by sleeping or even by taking a nap. These feelings can have a real impact on your life and how well you deal with things.

If you speak to general practitioners, they will tell you that there are many reasons behind people visiting surgeries regarding their sleep. Apart from the well-defined sleep disorders, people with depression might also consult their doctors because they are struggling with their sleep. Approximately 15 per cent of people diagnosed with depression sleep more than they want to. This then leads to more distress, which makes the feelings of depression worse. Some people also have obstructive sleep apnoea, caused by breathing difficulties while sleeping: you feel you have slept yet seem exhausted, really in need of more sleep. This is discussed further in Chapter 35.

That people oversleep may also be due to their socio-economic status: the greater their poverty, the less access to healthcare they have. Poorer people will be more likely to have an underlying condition that is undiagnosed and untreated, which may in turn cause more sleeping. Your sleep need may be increased because of short-term changes to your environment, such as when you have a new baby in the house. More long-term changes could also have a big impact, such as changing your job. There are also other possible reasons for 'oversleeping', including using alcohol or some other prescription drugs.

## Summary

There is no medical reason why increasing your sleep will lead to your needing even more sleep, but sleeping too much may be a symptom of some underlying health issue. What is important is recognizing, and taking, what sleep works for you – take how much you need.

## Top tips

1 Sleep for how long feels right for you. Ignore other people and anything you might hear or read that says to do otherwise.
2 Try to settle on a routine of sleeping the same, appropriate amount every night.
3 If you are worried, keep a sleep diary (see Chapter 1).

# 17

## 'Sleeping is a weakness'

Everything in moderation, including moderation.

Oscar Wilde, possibly

Sleeping is a weakness. This may seem an extreme viewpoint but the reality is that society takes this view. It revolves around the apparent contradiction between work and rest. The good worker, it is reasoned, needs to be at work, doing his or her job. Sleep interferes with this. The weakness is evident in performance at work, dedication, results and output. Indeed, there are well-known high-profile businesspeople who take pride in their short sleeping schedules.

This is what is known as a proxy, in that it is an estimate of the amount of time put into work, not a real measure of its quality. The amount of time at home asleep is an easy measure of time not at work, time not doing work, but the actual, more complex measures of output are harder to quantify.

I used to walk into work when I was doing my PhD. Arriving not much after 9 a.m., I would get a 'Good afternoon, Graham' from one of my colleagues. The greeting was designed to do two things: to criticize me and to make my colleague feel better. You can also call this sleep shaming, where the more you sleep, the more you are labelled as slacking off, not doing the job and not pulling your weight. Working isn't just about the time spent sitting at a desk, however; it's about what you produce at the end of each day, week, month and year.

This output is known as productivity, a measure of how much you produce, how much you create. It is a way to assess how much output you have been responsible for, regardless of the time and effort spent. Sleep contributes enormously to this; not in the way the sleep shamers mean but in how a lack of sleep can completely ruin your productivity.

## Less sleep is seen as a sign of a good worker

There are many phrases, sayings, adages that relate sleep to our strength and ability. There is a meme that reads: 'No one looks back on their life and remembers the nights they had plenty of sleep.' Sleep is seen as a time when we are vulnerable. Things may happen that we did not expect and cannot avoid. For example, Samson, the strong man in the Bible, lost his strength while he was asleep and his hair was cut off.

Many occupations see sleep as against the money-making values of the business. Long work hours are interrupted by the need to sleep. The former UK Prime Minister, Margaret Thatcher, famously was said to sleep very little, in the region of 4 hours per night. Her limited amount of sleep added to her mystique of strength, and her nickname 'the iron lady'. The less sleep/more work idea is taken to an extreme level in some societies. In Japan there is an officially recognized term, karoshi, which means 'overwork death', a diagnosis made when a person takes working hours to the extreme. This includes loss of sleep at a chronic level, leading to a heart attack or a stroke. The term was first reported in 1969 and is thought to contribute to many deaths each year.

It is interesting that before the European working time directive, junior doctors in the UK used to work an average of 70 hours per week. My wife did this for a few years and the tiredness got to the point where I had to pick her up from work because she was too tired to drive! Yet, bizarrely, the country thought that she could still save lives. These excessive working hours and lack of sleep can lead to mental health issues, sometimes resulting in suicide.

## Companies are making changes to encourage good sleep

Employers increasingly understand the need for members of staff to manage their work and non-work times. The work–life balance is essential. Some companies limit overtime; others go further, providing nap rooms and encouraging napping as a beneficial strategy for running their staff resources. In Japan, workers traditionally get less sleep on work nights than in other countries. Some firms are encouraging a nap on the job. Again in Japan there is something known as sleeping while present: having a nap at your desk, seated upright so as not to appear slovenly. There have been some calculations by economists, and it seems that by increasing productivity, each extra hour's sleep increases wages by nearly 5 per cent.

Shane and I have used the quote at the start of this chapter in one of our previous books. It is a good way to think about your whole life, a balance you should strive to achieve. Sleeping, resting is not a weakness – in fact quite the opposite. Too little sleep, insufficient balance, leads to weakness: weak minds, weak bodies, poor emotional strength. You make better decisions when you are fully rested, when exhaustion is not a factor.

## Summary

Traditionally a lack of sleep is seen as one way to represent strength, a hard worker, an important role model. These views are changing as society now recognizes the importance of sleep to maintain a high productivity. Many forward-thinking businesses are creating the environment and work culture to manage any lack of sleep and improve well-being, with the effect of improving the performance of their staff. Although society's attitude to sleep is gradually changing, there remains a section of it that still sees sleeping as a weakness.

## Top tips

1 If you are able, can you reduce the number of hours you sit at your desk? Can you improve your productivity by improving your sleep?
2 Can you look at taking a scheduled nap? This will improve your productivity after the nap.
3 Can you approach your employer to ask about the possibility of allowing an at-work nap? Be brave. The benefits should feed both ways: to you and to your employer.

# 18

# 'I can't sleep without my bed socks'

While asking people about their sleep, I have heard some curious and unusual ideas and myths, but this one seems completely mundane: socks; socks for bed. It first came about on a long-haul aeroplane flight, chatting with a lady who was not happy that we had been given no socks in our welcome pack. A first-world problem – she liked a pair of disposable socks, those very soft and loose articles along with the eye mask and the vomit bag.

Personally speaking I don't wear foot coverings when sleeping. I don't plan on over-sharing, but I go for the more natural sleeping cover – less is more. I think I may not be doing the same thing as everyone else, because I once saw a sign – from one of those shops selling non-products, with signs about everything and everyone – that said: 'Warm socks, good sleep.' Let's look at this.

## Your bedroom temperature is very important

You know that cold that seeps into your bones, when you don't feel you can warm up? If you feel this, a warm bath or shower before bed may be a good idea. Trying to fall asleep when you are very cold can be difficult, as we all know. When it is cold it is tempting to wear a pair of socks to bed; it is nice to have warm feet.

In colder climates there is a tendency to keep the bedroom very cold, perhaps as low as 10 °C. When my children went to nursery, for their afternoon nap they were tightly swaddled, put in a pram and left outside. Rain or shine, snow or fog. The boss of the nursery said they loved it – and they did sleep.

## The bedroom should not be too warm

Interestingly there are clear guidelines for regulating the temperature of a baby's bedroom. Babies seem to sleep best when their bedroom is between 16 and 20 °C (61–68 °F). Rather than trying to guess this temperature, you should use a room thermometer – they are cheap and easy to get hold of.

Regulating the heat or cold in your bedroom requires some effort. Your bedroom should be a few degrees cooler than the rest of the house. You may need to work more carefully with the radiator or heating controls. Consider thermostatic radiator valves to keep the heat stable. Invest in blinds and curtains, either warming or cooling. A fan can really help, which is something most people in more temperate climates only consider useful for a hot country.

The recommended range of temperatures for babies holds for grown-ups: again somewhere between 16 and 20 °C. As night wears on, your body naturally cools down, reducing your body temperature. You may have experienced that feeling when, on first getting into bed, it can feel too warm; you may then push your feet out from under the duvet or sheet, but, as time goes on and you feel cooler, you then pull the duvet closer. This should not come as a surprise: you are very still, your muscles are doing little work and not generating heat.

Some commentators ask you to think of your bedroom as a cave, presumably a little like a prehistoric human. Cool, dark and quiet. I'm not sure this helps much though. I have also seen someone writing that you should have a cool room and wear socks; this is described as being able to dilate your blood vessels faster. I am not sure what this really means, nor of any evidence that it works.

In previous scientific research that I conducted into radioactive gas in the air, called radon, a curious fact emerged. This gas is at very low concentrations and increases in concentration when we seal our houses with double glazing and draught proofing. In Scotland, however, there was a noticeable reduction in the gas levels. Anecdotally, it seems that many Scots leave their bedroom windows open at night, regardless of the temperature outside.

## A cool temperature is important to manage your sleep

The best thinking is that the room temperature will help your body to regulate your brain's temperature; it is set at a certain level for taking on sleep activity. It seems to affect most the rapid eye movement (REM) stage of sleep, the stage when you are likely to dream. Incidentally this seems to be a message that is heard in other cultures. I was chatting with a PhD student from Lebanon and she said there is this idea that if you sleep next to a heater it will give you bad dreams; and don't wear socks as this may make you suffocate. I don't know where to start with that one.

There is an added complexity: it seems that men and women are different in relation to their ideal room temperature. The evidence seems to rely on the resting metabolic rate of men and women. A woman has a metabolic activity that is lower than a man's, and this leads to less heat being generated. Therefore men may want a room slightly cooler than women. Nothing is straightforward.

## Summary

The temperature of your bedroom is very important for managing your sleep. If your bedroom is too cold it will be unpleasant and it may be difficult actually to fall asleep. However, it is straightforward to warm up, using duvets and warm clothing. One of the most common reasons for interfering with getting to sleep and staying asleep is that your bedroom is too warm. You may need to check the curtains or blinds and be aware of the level of heating in your bedroom, but, ultimately, socks may be useful.

## Top tips

1 Check the temperature of your bedroom using a room thermometer.
2 On hot days, keep windows shut and blinds and curtains closed until the outside temperature drops in the evening.
3 Think about using a thinner duvet when the temperatures are warm.
4 Wear socks if you are cold, if you are that way inclined.

# 19

# 'Napping is for old people'

As a society we sneer a little at people who take a nap during the day. It implies laziness, with images that come to mind of a senior citizen asleep in front of the television. This may be true to some extent, but it is not true that we should view it as a lazy thing to do.

If you sleep lightly and briefly, this is called a nap. Babies nap; they take short bursts of sleep, which lasts for a few years – babies and toddlers take a nap in the afternoon. Older people also often take a restorative nap during the day. Napping has a long history in society, and many famous people have been nappers, including John F. Kennedy and Albert Einstein.

Napping may be classified into three different types. The first is called planned or preparatory napping, which is when you take a nap before feeling sleepy. You may use this to prepare for an evening when you know you will not be able to have your usual sleep. An emergency nap happens when you cannot stay awake – you feel you have no choice. I certainly have that feeling, often when I know I have a few minutes to spare and think I could take 40 winks. This is what is recommended for people feeling drowsy while driving.

The third type is habitual napping, which is when you take a nap at the same time each day. This may coincide with a dip in your natural rhythms. It is a sort of nap that is very common after lunch, especially a big lunch. There are many cultures in the world that have a planned nap in this way, known as the siesta; it is a common practice across the countries that surround the Mediterranean. I've worked with a doctor from Italy who would have loved to have had a siesta after his big bowl of tagliatelle Bolognese, served up in our staff canteen, but, alas, he was usually denied this by a scheduled staff meeting.

## Benefits of a nap

Research into napping is gaining popularity, partly because it is something the policy makers feel could easily be implemented in a person's life. Speaking personally, napping research is great, because when I run a sleep lab during the daytime, it doesn't interfere with my night-time sleep. Very selfish I know.

The research going on at the moment shows that napping may be beneficial for a number of reasons. It improves your mood and it allows you to function more effectively. A nap, either planned or ad hoc, may also help to alleviate fatigue. A scientific paper looked at a nap and how frustrated and impulsive people felt afterwards. It found that they were less impulsive and better able to deal with frustrating events.

There is a strand of research looking at the effect of napping on chronic disorders such as diabetes, and on heart failure. This is potentially very exciting, and one we should all keep our eye on. Other more serious sleep disorders may also benefit from a nap. For example, narcolepsy, a debilitating disorder that causes the person to fall asleep at any time of the day, can be gently alleviated by a daytime nap or two. Scheduled napping may even be formally 'prescribed' by doctors to treat sleep disorders.

## The not-so-good news about napping

Despite some evidence showing that napping may be good for you, there is an equal and opposite interpretation of the research so far. This states that if you nap you are more likely to develop long-term chronic conditions. A nap isn't always the best thing for everyone. You may not be able to rest properly when you are not in your own bed. Lying on a couch or armchair may not allow rest to flow into a slumber. Some people may not be able to allow their midday dip to flow into a sleep.

The main issue with napping, at least in the short term, is that it may cause sleep inertia (see Chapter 4). This is the feeling of grogginess you have when you are not ready to take on the rest of your day. The short nap seems to be the most favoured intervention, but how do we define short? Most research defines a short nap as lasting 20–30 minutes. A study by NASA researchers, however, who put a lot of effort into working out how sleep affects their astronauts and pilots, found that a fairly long nap of 40 minutes increased performance by 34 per cent and alertness by 100 per cent.

It is important, first, to consider how you wake up: either feeling ready to go and enjoy the rest of the day or feeling groggy. The second issue is how much napping interferes with your night-time sleep. Can you still get to sleep in a reasonable time frame? Having a 2-hour nap may stop you from getting to sleep when you would normally. This can be very distressing and counterproductive.

The timing may also be important: you should leave enough time between waking and bedtime to allow a large enough sleep pressure to build up. Otherwise napping may interfere with your night-time sleep patterns and make it difficult to fall asleep at your regular bedtime.

## Working and alertness

You will be aware that there can be serious consequences to driving while sleepy. Sleep causes many road accidents, and government organizations work hard to try to reduce this. In the UK, the agency in charge of driving regulations, the Driver and Vehicle Licensing Agency (DVLA), has recently tightened its control of drivers – particularly commercial drivers – in relation to one specific issue, known as obstructive sleep apnoea. This is when you feel you slept all night but because of your throat closing up, the body has repeatedly woken up. This leads to extreme exhaustion and the fatigue leads to accidents. The overall advice remains that a short nap is recommended for those who feel their concentration is wandering.

Other issues with sleep arise from shift work. A short nap and caffeine afterwards are recommended to alleviate tiredness and improve productivity. Some workplaces are bringing in a dedicated room, a 'nap room', designed to allow members of staff to take a short rest. This obviously relies on trust, but when it works, it can have enormous benefits for productivity. This would be, for a sleep evangelist such as myself, a brilliant and very positive change to working practices.

## Summary

Taking a nap during the day has a long history but it remains a practice sneered at by some in society. A good napping schedule may help you enormously to alleviate fatigue and improve your productivity. Some forward-thinking employers are introducing short naps during the working day to help keep members of staff working to their maximum capability.

## Top tips

1 Do you nap regularly? If you have excessive daytime sleepiness, you may need to check for an underlying sleep disorder such as obstructive sleep apnoea.
2 A scheduled nap may help you be more productive, more alert, more creative.
3 Keep a nap short, something like 10–20 minutes. Aim to take this in the early afternoon – no later in the day so as to not interfere with your evening sleep.

# 20

# 'One hour's sleep before midnight is worth two after'

One hour before midnight is worth two after.

Mrs Iris Murphy, Graham's grandma, 1971 to present

My grandma used to say that every hour spent asleep before midnight was worth two after midnight. She also used to say 'You can go off people, you know', but that's a different conversation. This bedtime advice all sounded like a ploy to get me to go to bed earlier, and probably happens in many homes, but many people ask me if this is true, so it feels like a myth worth exploring.

So the premise is that if you go to bed after midnight, you are going to have to catch up on your sleep by sleeping extra hours in the morning, more than you would normally. We need to explore how the body governs itself, particularly in relation to the time of day and night. The actual time that the clock points at is not really important. The numbers are merely a way of describing the actual phase you are in in the 24-hour day. The time will vary by place on the Earth and the time of year. Instead of thinking about the time in an absolute sense, we need to think about how the body governs itself.

## Your body is able to keep track of your environment

Your body is amazing, for loads of reasons, and one is how you work with the Earth's movement. You detect light and dark, use food cues, social interactions, and these routines all interact with your genes. These genetic codes are in every cell in your body and they define your metabolism over a 24-hour day. Your eyes are detecting light all the time, even while you are asleep, and information on the amount of light is constantly being passed to your brain. This allows your metabolism, particularly your hormones, to fiddle unconsciously with your rhythms, keeping you in balance with your environment.

Modern life, electric lighting, long evenings socializing are all different from what our predecessors' bodies experienced for millions of years. We have evolved to work with our environment. To some extent we have been able to break the hold the natural environment had over us, but this is not necessarily a good thing for our health.

Having a time to go to bed that is past when the sun drops below the horizon, enjoying our new-found ability not to be governed by the sun and the moon, may lead to difficulties. Bearing in mind how quickly we have changed our world, it is amazing that we have been able to deal with this. The evidence is, however, that a later bedtime may not be good for our health, even if we can still operate to the best of our abilities.

## Your sleep has distinct stages

Most of you will take to your bed in a fairly regular manner at some point between 9 p.m. and midnight. If you then choose to stay awake past your normal bedtime, the body has to decide what to do. It may choose to be ready to react, making wakefulness important to avoid danger. Although it is unlikely that you'll be facing a scary foe, there are consequences for your sleep. That said, there is no science behind the idea that every hour spent asleep before midnight is worth two after midnight – an old grandmother's tale, or at least one from my grandma.

A further issue is that the early part of your sleep in the night is very important, where much of the deep sleep – what we scientists call slow-wave sleep – happens. Disrupting this time may not allow you to feel fully refreshed for the following day. Sleep occurs in stages, which go through cycles of light sleep to deep sleep, then rapid eye movement (REM) sleep and back to light sleep. These cycles go on throughout the night of sleep, but the first two or three contain significant amounts of slow-wave sleep, the deep sleep. Each cycle lasts something like 60–90 minutes, and the first 4 hours are key. These then define a core sleep, an absolutely essential time frame for healthy functioning.

I was never too sure about these cycles. How can the most deep sleep happen in the first 4 hours of slumber? Surely your body would reward you more when you sleep for a long time. When I analyse the output from my study participants' brain scans in my laboratory, however, I can see clearly that this is what happens. It seems counterintuitive.

## Deep sleep is important for your health

The deep-sleep stage is very important for a variety of reasons only now starting to become apparent. There is a clear need for this stage in your sleep, as it helps lay down memories on how to do things, such as learning new skills and memorizing information. It also helps to reset your body and your metabolism, and to lower levels of the stress hormone cortisol. Your nervous system is also active during this stage as your body strives to consolidate the activities of the daytime and prepare you for the next day.

There is also a more obvious reason why getting sleep before midnight may be important. You are governed by the real clock also, not just your internal body clock. So if you go to bed late at night and you have an alarm set, you will simply have less time to sleep. We don't often allow ourselves to wake when we want to, when our body naturally feels like it is ready for the day. This inevitable reduction in time in bed will have a knock-on effect.

## Summary

The myth that going to sleep before midnight may be important has some basis in truth. Your body needs the early sleep to benefit from the deep-sleep stage. Without this, your body is unable to operate in a healthy way. The exact number of hours' improvement will be highly dependent on the individual, but nevertheless there is some clear benefit from going to bed earlier.

## Top tips

1 Think about going to bed a little earlier than normal. Don't allow this to leave you tossing and turning in bed, but try to set your bedtime nice and early.

2 Don't be tempted to leave insufficient time for a good sleep. You can always catch up with the television or finish your book tomorrow!

# 21

# 'I just need an app'

Do you have a smartphone? I was first introduced to them by my brother-in-law. He wanted to show me these new-fangled apps, and he had chosen a fishing game for the introduction. As you could imagine, we spent a few minutes 'throwing' the line to catch the next trout.

This game was a little limited but it showed a very important component of this gadget: an accelerometer. It measures, as its name suggests, the acceleration – essentially, the movement – of the gadget. Accelerometers are built into many things and have given rise to a new class of product. These are the little pieces of equipment that you wear to tell you how much effort you are putting in, how many steps you've taken, even how many calories you've burned.

## There are devices for measuring your activity and your sleep

As the opposite of activity is stillness, which does occur when you are asleep, devices such as pedometers use the cessation of activity, or stillness, to indicate sleep. There are also many smartphone apps that claim to do myriad different tasks, including measuring your sleep. Some link to the sleep pattern and the time of night, using your preferred wake-up time somehow to manage your wake-up so as to prevent grogginess. Some even claim to be able to work out the amount of time you spent in each stage of sleep, to know if you are in rapid eye movement (REM) sleep and even when you are in slow-wave deep sleep. It is probably wise to approach these claims with some scepticism.

Once again it is necessary to stress that we are all different and have different levels of movement and activity as we sleep. The only correct method to work out the different stages of your sleep is to use a sensor on the scalp, which measures the electrical activity in your brain.

Perhaps we will soon be able to link a sensor placed on the scalp wirelessly to our phones to measure our sleep more accurately. There have been some start-up companies that have done this but none has made a success of it. It is probably only a matter of time before someone manages to do so.

## Accelerometers are used in research

Many scientific research projects into sleep have measured activity using an accelerometer. There are so many things to work through to see if these are a useful tool, such as how many nights to wear the accelerometer for, where on the body to attach it and how to summarize the data into something useful.

Some of the research suggests that, during sleep, the device overestimates an adult's sleep and underestimates a child's. This is probably because of how fidgety kids can be – the device thinks they are awake and moving.

There are other obvious reasons for underestimating the time asleep. This may be due to having a sleep disorder whereby your body is not completely still while you sleep. One such condition that affects many people is periodic limb movement disorder, in which your body repeatedly moves (often it is the legs), which would make your device think you were awake.

## Summary

These devices may be useful for large-scale studies and for measuring activity rather than sleep. They are probably not overly useful for assessing your sleep at present, but may be in the future.

## Top tips

1 If you have an app or a device to measure your sleep, use it with caution.
2 Use a sleep diary (see Chapter 1) to give you an idea of how much you feel you sleep, and compare it to the information gained from your app.

# 22

# 'My baby doesn't "sleep like a baby"!'

Having a child is amazing – a life-changing event, and exhausting. This book cannot deal with sleep for a baby or infant in a comprehensive way: there are plenty of other books on that subject. Shane will examine some types of behaviours, which include both the things we do and our thoughts that influence sleep. For example, our expectations can make it more or less likely that we get to sleep. As is the case with adults, it is important for children to learn a schedule for sleep. It is through making these associations that they learn how to go to sleep and, consequently, we get good sleep, too.

## Is there a problem?

The starting point must be identifying whether or not your child has any issue relating to sleep. There are all sorts of facts and schedules regarding the amount of time your child should sleep, but it does not seem necessary to offer them here. If there is some difficulty regarding your child's sleep or crying during the night, then we can pretty safely say that this will be an issue for you as a parent.

This does not, however, mean there is an underlying sleep disorder or an organic cause for your child's behaviour. 'Organic' refers to a cause from a physical or physiological issue. As a general guide, after the birth of your child, it takes about 3 to 6 months for an infant to sleep through the night. If this has been delayed, then it is worth consulting with your general practitioner regarding gaining extra support and help with sleep issues. There are also some great, locally run voluntary sector organizations that may be able to help.

A good sleeper does not equal a good baby. As a psychologist, Shane aims to be non-judgemental. Taking a non-judgemental stance is important for a successful outcome with therapy. As in the chapter on mindfulness (see Chapter 7), when dealing with your child's sleep issues, try not to evaluate the child him or herself, and do this by taking a non-judgemental stance. Bring your attention to what is happening as opposed to factors that are good or indeed bad. Often our opinions get in the way of the facts.

## Co-sleeping with your infant

It is fairly common for parents to sleep, or doze, with their baby or infant in bed with them. This can be a strategy for getting some sleep, especially when breastfeeding, but there are concerns about it because an association has been discovered between this practice and Sudden Infant Death Syndrome.

There is some helpful guidance from the UK government in relation to sleep safety. Ensure your baby cannot fall out of the bed or become trapped, particularly against a wall. Maintaining a cool temperature is important, so be aware of the heat you are both generating (see Chapter 18). Use sheets and do not cover your child's head. Of course, the usual advice of putting babies to bed on their backs also applies when co-sharing. Also, although this seems obvious, remember that babies should not have a pillow for their first year, and this applies wherever they sleep, including in your bed.

As with adults, improving the sleep hygiene behaviours of your child is an important first step. Things that get in the way of, or contaminate, the association between bed and sleep are behaviours that are within your control. As with adults, there are normal waking cycles in the night, and just because your child wakes does not mean you have to comfort him or her, or to intervene. As you become more attuned to your child, you will identify crying that has a particular meaning, such as a cry identifiable as signalling hunger.

In attempting to solve your child's difficulties with sleep, it is important to focus on the facts and identify what the cause is. For example, the child may be unable to fall asleep except while being held. In this case the child has never learned to fall asleep alone, and the goal is to learn this skill and become more resilient, over time, to more disruption and change. As with managing anxiety, it is important to expect some resistance and difficulty in this new learning period. You should expect some crying, possibly from you and your baby.

## We need to establish a set of conditions at bedtime

What we wish to achieve is a gradual change in the child's behaviour if a sleep issue is present. This can be achieved by increasing the time between when you put your child down to sleep and when you respond to your child crying. This is often referred to as controlled crying. On the first day of attempting to help your child fall asleep, it might be useful to start by waiting 5 minutes before responding. Then increase this to 10 minutes and then 15 minutes before you return to the crying child. On the second day, you can progressively increase this, first by waiting 10 minutes and then 15 and then 20 minutes before returning. This gives your child an opportunity to increase his or her ability to cope with your being outside the room but also to get better at sleeping alone. Your child gets more and more time to practise getting to sleep without you present.

## Possible organic causes of poor sleep

There are several possible medical conditions that may have an impact on a child's sleep. These include colic, a catch-all term for a child crying very often and being difficult to calm. Other chronic illnesses such as asthma may also affect a child's ability to sleep. Any possible causes that are worrying you are best ruled out by a visit to your general practitioner.

## Summary

Your baby needs to learn how and when to sleep, which may take some effort on your part. First of all you must rule out any physical issues for your baby. Then you can adopt a strategy that fits with you and your parenting style. Also, finally, be aware of the safety of your child if you share a bed.

## Top tips

1 First of all, try to rule out there being any possible medical cause of your child's difficulties with getting to sleep .
2 Be careful when co-sharing a bed – check through the issues for safety in this chapter.
3 Take time to work out the strategy that you feel happy with and then persevere.
4 Don't lose heart, it is difficult and it will pass.

# 23

# 'Cheese gives you nightmares'

Dreams are not sent by God.

Aristotle, 'On Prophesying by Dreams'

Are you running away from someone? He is catching up with you, but your feet cannot move fast enough. You feel as though you are jelly; your legs and feet are useless. I bet you've experienced a nightmare; people can report at least once in their lives when they woke sweating, heart racing, distressed by really vivid events in a dream. I have found – based on absolutely no science – that I have vivid dreams after eating cheese before bedtime. So I hope this is true rather than a myth. Weirdly, last night I had some cheese on toast before bed, and I had a bizarre set of dreams. Not nightmares exactly, but a retelling of the television crime series I had been watching. It seems the right time for me to look into whether or not cheese gives us nightmares.

The best scientific evidence we have at the moment is that dreams, and therefore nightmares, happen during rapid eye movement (REM) sleep. This is a particular stage of sleep that happens more during the second part of the sleep. The first half has less REM activity. During our sleep we have what is known as sleep paralysis: we are unable to move our arms and legs normally during this time. Your body is amazing: it seems that you would act out your dreams if your body were able to move. Your brain makes sure this does not happen during a nightmare.

## Dreams may be triggered by stressful events

I must stress that I have no research interest in dreams, nor in the spiritual significance they hold for some people. Shane treats people with post-traumatic stress disorder (PTSD), which has at its heart the re-experiencing of a traumatic event. A traumatic event can change a belief about yourself, the world, other people

74

or indeed your future, and nightmares are ways these beliefs can surface. Memories of the trauma can be re-experienced in a nightmare. As the founding psychoanalyst Sigmund Freud identified, in our dreams we do not censor information, so individuals with PTSD often experience repeated, disturbing dreams of a stressful experience. However, this is not to suggest that all dreams are a result of stressful events; in fact many dreams are a pleasant experience. We all accept that dreams happen, but can eating cheese be a trigger?

## Studies of cheese and nightmares

One of the earlier real studies of this phenomenon was carried out by the British Cheese Board. In this study, 200 people were given 20 g (a little under three-quarters of an ounce) of cheese 30 minutes before bed. They were then asked to describe any dreams or nightmares they had. However, to make this more interesting the researchers used different types of cheese. This study was not published, nor peer-reviewed, but it did provide some entertaining conclusions.

Two-thirds of those participating reported a dream. They found that Cheddar cheese tended to produce dreams about celebrities, Red Leicester nostalgic dreams often related to childhood. Cheese from Lancashire produced dreams about work, which could arguably be termed a nightmare for some people. Stilton cheese seemed to be related to the most vivid, unusual and downright strange dreams. Cheshire cheese gave peaceful sleep, without dreams. Nice.

The study stated that there are high levels of tryptophan in cheese, which is known to be involved in the production of melatonin, a major sleep hormone. Their studies were not designed with a placebo group, however, and therefore would not be well respected in the scientific world.

In 2015, a study entitled 'Dreams of a rarebit fiend' was published in the psychology journal *Frontiers in Psychology*. The authors interviewed 396 students about their perceptions regarding what they eat and how they dream. They found that 18 per cent said they had more vivid or disturbing dreams after eating food. The foods most likely to evoke dreams were dairy products, such as cheese. As an aside, these authors also found that spicy foods led to particularly disturbing dreams.

## Possible causes of dreaming after cheese

There are many proposed hypotheses as to why sleep and dreaming may be affected by cheese, or food in general. There have been some rumblings about how the bacterial and fungal content of cheese produces psychoactive toxins that will then cause us to dream. There seem to be three other explanations. The first is that there may be a link between being sensitive to dreams and eating specific foods, particularly dairy foods. A second hypothesis is that a general change in your body's state, caused by eating food generally, may lead to dreaming. This has links back to antiquity: the Ancient Greek physician Hippocrates apparently believed that adverse reactions to food could lead to bizarre dreams. Changes particularly in the gut seem to be associated with disruption of sleep, which may cause a change in dreaming. The third hypothesis is based on our prior beliefs: we hear a sleep myth and believe that happens then to us; this is known as the folklore hypothesis.

The fact is that only a rigorous scientific study will discover whether or not there truly is a link between what we eat – particularly close to bedtime – and the dreams we have.

I often do seem to have a vivid dream the night after eating cheese, but, speaking as a scientist, this feels like what is known as confirmation bias. This means that we tend to give more credibility to a situation that agrees with what we believe may be true.

## Summary

Food may have an impact on sleep, although it may be that cheese does not lead to nightmares. If you find that certain types of food at night – be these cheese or hot spicy foods or even certain drinks – cause distressing dreams or other symptoms, then consider excluding these from your diet for a while and see what happens.

## Top tips

1 Do you wake in the night, feeling uncomfortable? Do you get reflux, heartburn? Think about your diet, particularly in the evening.

2 Consider cutting from your diet foods you suspect may be having an impact on the quality of your sleep, particularly spicy and fat-laden foods.

# 24

## 'There must be something wrong with me if I sleep more than my friends'

General practitioners who are friends of mine report that it is common for people to come to see them with worries caused by comparing their sleep with how they think others sleep, convinced a medical condition must be causing their need to sleep longer than others. Perhaps they are fed up with being called lazy because of the length of time they spend asleep. When the examination and blood tests turn out to be normal, what then is the cause?

First of all, you are a unique individual. Your sleep needs are for you only, and you should not listen to others. If you are concerned about the amount of time you sleep, or are just curious, record how much you sleep each night. Write down when you fall asleep and when you wake up. Keep the sleep diary for a week (see Chapter 1). This will allow you to work out what your patterns of sleep are. These are your patterns, not someone else's.

Then when you have done this, take a look at your results. Trust your mind when making decisions. Remember that your sleep can be as long or as short as you need. The key is that you do not have excessive tiredness during the daytime. If you like to sleep for 10 hours, then that is your decision; and if you sleep for 5 hours and feel great, then that is right for you. Don't listen to any criticisms from other people. They may just be envious!

The Japanese writer Haruki Murakami is known for keeping a strict sleep routine of going to bed at 9 p.m. and waking at 4 a.m. It works for him, and he said: 'I keep to this routine every day without variation. The repetition itself becomes the important thing; it's a form of mesmerism. I mesmerize myself to reach a deeper state of mind.'

The worst thing you can do is become stressed over the amount of sleep you get. If it works for you then that is your perfect amount. Do not feel under pressure to conform, especially since, as already explained, sleep does not often take place in 'natural' conditions any more. Remember that with the advent of lighting, night-time became a time during which you could be productive. People became sensitive to being 'efficient' with their time and 'productive' during darkness. Don't be tempted, however, to sacrifice your well-being in order to increase your level of activity or strive to achieve a greater number of things.

## You need what you need

What does this tell us about the amount of sleep we should be getting? Well, the advice is that you need what you need, a little like a famous story from Zen Buddhism, when a student of Zen asked his teacher: 'Master, what is enlightenment?' The master replied: 'When hungry, eat. When tired, sleep.' A little extreme, but the point is that you should rest when you need to. You should not sleep for 8 hours if your body is telling you that you need fewer or more.

Here are some ways of checking what you need.

1 How long does it take you to fall asleep? This period is known as sleep onset latency by sleep scientists; it should last around 10–20 minutes before you are asleep. If you are taking more time than this, it is one way of your body saying it is not ready for sleep. Conversely, if you fall asleep as soon as your head hits the pillow, you are perhaps waiting too long before going to bed.

2 Do you wake up before your alarm? This may be your brain's way of telling you that you have had enough sleep. You should not feel under pressure to go back to sleep just to fit in with your alarm. Remember that an alarm is an unnatural way to manage your sleep. People have reported improvements in sleep when they stopped being tied to an alarm.

3 How do you feel during the day? Daytime sleepiness contributes to low levels of well-being. Everyone has times of feeling tired or sleepy. That is entirely reasonable. If you feel the urge to fall asleep while you are eating your lunch or reading a book in the evening, though, this may be more problematic. Conversely, if

you don't feel this way, then the sleep you are getting is probably just right for you.

## Summary

This chapter has reiterated some important messages. Sleep is not a competition; there is no need to be better at it than anyone else. Your sleep habits are about you and your well-being, and don't let anyone tell you otherwise.

## Top tips

1 Accept your sleep habits and don't compare yourself to others unfavourably. When you learn to accept what your body needs, sleep will become easier for you.

2 Don't forget that the amount of sleep varies at different times in your life. Don't compare your current sleep need with those of a former you. Again, accepting this will improve your sleep. Time spent thinking 'I used to need only 7 hours. Why do I now need more?' isn't helpful and is likely to affect your ability to drop off.

# 25

# 'When I exercise, I sleep better'

Exercise requires physical effort; it does have a purpose. The aim of exercise is to maintain or improve your health and fitness. This can be mental health or physical health. Exercise prevents physical illnesses – such as heart and lung diseases, high blood pressure, diabetes, obesity, cancer, dementia, Alzheimer's disease and Parkinson's disease – while also managing mental health issues such as anxiety, depression and high levels of stress. There is also an important aspect of exercise that is often glossed over: it may be an important social event for you. This should be factored into your week, as social events are also good cues for your own body clock.

While looking at the research on exercise and sleep I had to chuckle to myself. A recent scientific research project said that you will need to exercise for at least 4 months before it will have a positive impact on your sleep. One newspaper expressed clear disappointment that it would take so much time and so much effort. This epitomizes one of the negative aspects with modern society: we expect instant results with minimal effort.

## Type of exercise is important

A number of research projects have looked at sleep in relation to exercise. One of these was able to show that moderate exercise could help alleviate the symptoms of chronic insomnia – in this particular project, moderate exercise related to walking for a short period of time, such as 20 minutes per day. These efforts reduced the time it took to fall asleep and increased the length of time asleep during the night. Sounds perfectly intuitive.

However, the same study showed that high intensity exercise, such as lifting weights, was unable to improve insomnia. So the effect of exercise on sleep may be dependent on exactly what form of exercise you do. You cannot do one session of exercise and expect instant results. It requires effort over at least 16 weeks before consistent improvement will be shown. The mechanism that leads to exercise improving sleep is unknown. It may be due to the changes in body temperature that you experience while exercising and after you stop and rest, but just as likely is the effect exercise can have on your mood, on levels of anxiety and feelings of stress and depression.

## How much do you need?

The amount of exercise may also play a part. The research suggests the ideal is 150 minutes' exercise per week, which most people should find easy to incorporate into their daily agendas. Those who did, showed a 65 per cent increase in sleep quality, with a reduction in daytime sleepiness. Of course, you are probably aware of the benefits of exercise on your cardiac health and blood sugar control. Also that it has an impact on your ability to stay slim and your joints working properly. It now seems that, in addition, it improves the quality of your sleep.

## When should you exercise?

The timing of your exercise routine seems to play a part in how it affects sleep. Afternoons seem a good time for your workout, mornings less so. Experts have settled on the ideal time for a workout being approximately 6 hours before you go to sleep. Also, avoid exercise, particularly high-intensity exercise, in the few hours before you go to bed and to sleep. Otherwise this seems to work your body rhythm into a higher level, which is not conducive to sleep.

If you exercise too late it may be difficult to fall asleep. It is likely that this is because of the increases in the hormones adrenalin and cortisol. Adrenalin is the 'fight or flight' hormone response, designed for survival in trying and dangerous circumstances. These hormones make it obvious to your body that sleep is not on the agenda. This may mean that daytime exercise is better preparation for night-time sleep than the evening run around a hockey pitch. Daytime light is also important for setting your body clock, so you know it is daytime and your body should be doing daytime activities. This will mean heading outside, which is easier said than done during a long, cold winter.

This view, however, remains contentious, as some studies have found that evening exercise may be beneficial. We return to the old adage of individual preference. You should try it, see what happens, see what works for you, and then make a decision.

Again speaking from personal experience, yoga and relaxation in the evening do not interfere with my sleep. I have done Sivananda yoga for many years, stretching, twisting, strengthening mind, body and emotions. This takes effort and hard work and I have thought about stopping many times; I am very lucky – my wife joins me and she 'encourages' me to keep going. After the 75-minute session, I remain awake for about another 2 hours and then fall fast asleep, happy with my success on my yoga mat.

## Summary

Stating that exercise is good for you seems to be a common feature of so many self-help texts. Well, I won't disappoint you. Looking in detail at the evidence around this myth, I would support it as being true in connection with sleep. It is not a blanket 'non-stop exercise at any time of the day', but subtler than that. Choose your time and choose the intensity. I am also biased, but I strongly urge you to try a gentle, strengthening regime such as yoga or Pilates.

## Top tips

1 Do at least 2.5 hours' moderate-level exercise per week.
2 Choose the time of day carefully. Try to finish at least 2–3 hours before bedtime.
3 Consider restricting high-intensity exercise to daytime.

# 26

# 'Teenagers are lazy because they sleep too much'

Teenagers have only two friends: everyone and no one. I heard this when my kids were approaching their teenage years, but I didn't understand what it meant. I do now! Let me explain. The media, and friends and family, often complain that teenagers can sleep all morning, especially during the holidays, and getting them up in the morning can indeed be a terrible battle. It turns out – well, so I'm reliably informed by my teenage daughters – that 'Everyone stays up late, Dad' and 'No one goes to bed before midnight, Dad.' Who'd have known?

There is more to this than some problem we have with our next generation, though. Being a teenager is an important part of growing up; it is a critical job each of us must do. It is also one of the most exciting parts of your life; you are learning, developing, growing up. You are forming friendships, romantic liaisons. It is exciting.

Let's deal with some myths as we discuss teenage machinations. Western society has the idea that those who wake early are hard working and probably clever. This comes in part from hearing about how well some societies are doing with academic subjects, such as in the Chinese model of teaching. This includes early starts and long days.

## Insufficient sleep has some worrying outcomes for teens

A large national survey in the USA, known as the Youth Risk Behavior Survey, found that in 2007, only 31 per cent of high-school students got 8 or more hours' sleep. In just 8 years, this has dropped to 27 per cent in 2015. The USA has set an objective to increase the proportion of teens sleeping 8 or more hours to around one-third.

Teens' physical health is, on the whole, going to be good and unaffected by poor sleep. Short-term tiredness and exhaustion may happen, but can be remedied by some catch-up sleep. Of course, this is a challenging time, with hormones causing the physical, mental and emotional changes during puberty; this may also have an impact on sleep.

There may also be issues with behaviour that are directly caused by lack of sleep. These adverse behaviours may range from the mildly antisocial all the way through to taking part in crime. The main reason we become concerned about poor sleep in the teenage years is that we expect our youngsters to be learning. It is the most productive phase for learning about languages, sciences, mathematics, history and the arts.

Critical in this learning process is sleep. Many studies have shown that obtaining sleep, particularly the deepest stage of sleep known as slow-wave sleep, is critical for learning. One scientific theory is that sleep helps us to consolidate memories: what we have been taught during the day can be laid down as long-term memory during sleep. This has been shown when people sleep after learning, and this includes naps during the daytime. We really don't know how this process works. There is growing evidence that a cleaning process during sleep strengthens the nerve connections within our brain. This also frees up space for another day of learning. This freeing of space may explain why, if you miss a night's slumber, you will find it much more difficult to learn anything the next day.

Also, growing evidence suggests that the rapid eye movement (REM) stage of sleep is important for processing perception and emotional experiences. This is likely to help maintain a good, positive mood, able to deal with stress. The second half of your sleep is when you take most REM sleep. Missing this latter stage of your sleep pattern may have effects on your emotional and mental health.

As so often happens, we must return to our biological clock: the circadian rhythm (see Chapter 15). This is critical for our well-being, learning and health. As you might imagine, these rhythms exist for all of us, at any age, but they are not fixed, as we see only too well with babies. A newborn imposes a simple system of eating and sleeping throughout the 24-hour day. This is so different from an adult's rhythm and so it is that parents' tiredness ensues (see Chapter 22).

It should not come as a surprise, then, that teenagers also have different rhythms from adults. Adolescents become sleepier later on in the evening. They also need an hour or so more sleep, in an ideal world. They have to contend, however, with the hopes and aspirations of parents and teachers, with the fixed schedule of the school day. This is then compounded by poor sleep hygiene – and maybe poor hygiene, but that is a different subject. Smartphones, gadgets, light-emitting objects all interfere with the natural rhythms. Combine this with late-night parties at weekends, and it is surprising we make it through this period at all.

## The school day starts early

You probably subscribe to the idea that a good night's sleep will lead to better health and this is the same for teenagers. There is a contradiction that society has imposed on our future minds, however, by setting up an early start to their day. Research has shown that the later young adults start their school day, the better their results. In fact, a paper with the snappy title 'A's from zzzz's', written by two economists, found that a 50-minute later start time is equivalent to improving a teacher's ability to get good results by over 30 per cent above the average. Other studies have estimated an improvement, from a 1-hour delay to school start time, in terms of an 8 per cent increase in future earnings or being equivalent to having one-third fewer students in each class.

A research article that used the best scientific method for summarizing all the research, known as a systematic review, showed that delayed start times for school increased the total amount of sleep. Well done, Sherlock! It also showed, however, that there was better performance in terms of thinking and learning, academic results and improvements in mood. What should we do? There are research projects being conducted right now in which the start time for school is 1 hour later, put back to 10 a.m. instead of 9 a.m. for those teenagers doing their first set of really important exams. We eagerly await the results, but, meanwhile, you should encourage teenagers to sleep for 9 hours, or more, each night.

## Good sleep habits last a lifetime

When I asked my youngest daughter what she thought about sleep in teenagers, she replied: 'It's great, so kids sleep.' I think this shows that teenagers get its importance, but do not always get sufficient sleep. This is for specific reasons. Bedtime is later in teenagers, as it seems the hormone melatonin is secreted later in the day and this controls sleepiness. Also, in the morning, it lasts longer than it does in adults, making it harder for teenagers to wake up. Their brains are going through as much change as newborns, so it is understandable that they need to recover. That does not stop it from frustrating parents, but, as teenagers move into their twenties, a more standard amount of time asleep establishes – usually 7–9 hours.

Remember that habits learned in adolescence often become lifetime habits, so make sure they learn good sleep habits early and they'll last a lifetime. Recently the American Academy of Sleep Medicine recommended teenagers should try to achieve 8–10 hours' sleep per night, every night.

## Summary

The evidence seems to disprove this chapter's myth. The fact is that teenagers need more sleep than adults – this is really important for their normal development and learning. The evidence also shows that, far from sleeping too much, most teenagers do not sleep enough. Their sleep patterns are different from adults' and we need to respect this. We must hope that the current research looking at changing the school day will help here.

## Top tips

1 In terms of improving sleep, this chapter only applies to you personally if you are a teenager. Ask your parents to read it in the hope that they will understand you better and not expect you to sleep the same as they do. Unfortunately, unless you are in a school with start times that suit your sleep patterns, you will have no choice but to conform on weekdays. Fortunately, though, it seems that teenagers are good at catching up on lost sleep, so you can make up for it at the weekend.

2 If you are a parent of teenagers, let them sleep if they need to sleep – it's not laziness, it is physiological. You can encourage them to improve their sleep using techniques described in this book, but do not expect the result to be that they sleep at the same times you do. As we have seen, sleep habits acquired in adolescence persist into adulthood, so it is beneficial to get into good habits young.

# 27

## 'You shouldn't keep your mobile phone by your bed'

There has been a real change in the Western world, a recent development that has relied on some amazing technological innovations. We now have this amazing gadget, like something out of a science fiction television programme – think *Star Trek* or *Blake's 7*. A small piece of plastic that can attach you to a world of knowledge, all the friends you ever wanted, a future romantic partner. It comes at a cost, though. All these devices shine light out, be they mobile phones, smartphones, tablets, laptops, desktop computers or backlit eBooks. They project electromagnetic radiation, which you can distinguish as a different-coloured light, into your eyes.

Why is this harmful? We are surrounded by light all day. Our bodies use this important environmental cue to keep on track – a process known as entrainment. The thing is, for most of human history, we operated on sunlight only. Sometimes this may be reflected from the moon, but the sun remains the source of light. We have now changed, and this has many consequences.

### Light at night may disrupt your sleep

This has nothing to do with a difficulty astronomers have with light pollution, which is when the night sky cannot be seen properly as a result of the artificial light coming from street lights and so on, especially near built-up areas and our cities. Rather, the difficulty here is that your eyes, detecting light at night, pass the information on to your brain which reacts accordingly.

This is particularly important when it comes down to the colour of the light. Sunlight, and all light we use to illuminate our world, is constructed from a series of wavelengths, which we detect as different colours. The wavelength that we see as blue is detected by more than the cells you use to see.

In addition to the cells you learned about in a biology lesson at school, there is a class of cells, discovered during the 1990s, known as the photosensitive ganglion cells. You cannot see with these cells – that is, they do not provide you with visual information – but they do support your body's circadian rhythm (see Chapter 15). They pass information to a part of your brain known as the supra-chiasmatic nucleus, and the body then assumes that you should be wide awake. This is good during the day but not at night. Your eyes should be seeing far less light, at much lower strengths.

Blue light causes your body to suppress production of melatonin, an essential hormone that causes your body to enter a resting state ready for sleep. Your eyes are very sensitive to blue light. This suppression will make your body feel awake, and it also raises your heart rate.

Blue light comes from many devices, so if you use your smart-phone late in the evening, this will suppress melatonin production and, in turn, your body will not relax, ready to sleep. It seems the more passive devices, such as some eBooks that are not backlit, are more similar to a traditional paper book and so do not interfere with the circadian rhythm in this way. These use whatever light is on in your surroundings to light up the display rather than emit-ting light themselves.

## Lack of light in the day may also disrupt sleep

Although what has been said above may lead you to think that blue light is problematic, it is also very important. Light during the day is needed to direct your body to understand that it is daytime (entrainment). If you do not get blue light in the day, you may start to produce the sleep hormone melatonin.

To look at this, scientists conducted a study, exposing people to different levels of light during the day. They found that those who were not exposed to daylight were sleepier during the day than those who were and this lack of daylight messed with their normal rhythms. The advice is that you should go out into sunshine or at least light in the day so that your body stays on track.

A sad consequence of ageing is that the lenses in our eyes become yellowed. This has a knock-on effect for perceiving blue light in the day – it reduces its intensity. A cataract can cut down the level of light we receive even more. These may provide some answers to the question, why does our sleep change as we get older?

## Mental activity may not help you relax

The modern world has become fairly obsessed with communication. Most people have a phone or other device on all day and all night, constantly waiting for a message, a new photograph, some gossip or a new cute cat photograph. I have spoken with many people who insist that it is essential they have their phone by their bed, just in case someone needs to contact them in the night. A recent study found that a third of adults look at their smartphones during the night when they should be asleep.

People seem to think that it is all right for a smartphone, or other similar device, to be left at their bedside all night. Indeed, now that the initial concerns about brain tumours from radiation have receded, this has become a common practice, especially among young people.

They think it is a good way to relax. Not so. These devices contain work; they house mental activity and, often, distressing events, too. These all make it more difficult for you to relax and nod off. A classic reason for finding it difficult to fall asleep at bedtime – or, indeed, to go back to sleep after waking during the night – is thinking. Thinking keeps your mind active; it will not allow the hormones to seep into your brain cells, relax your muscles, allow you freedom from the daytime.

## There are ways to change

As you can imagine, manufacturers are finding solutions to these issues. There is software you can install to suppress the blue light emitted from a computer or smartphone screen.

An alternative solution that may work is wearing yellow-tinted sunglasses at night to avoid the blue wavelengths, ensuring that you will become naturally tired, which may help induce sleep more quickly. Otherwise, consider leaving your phone in the living room, not next to your bed. The world will not fall apart if you have not looked at Facebook.

## Summary

It would appear that the advice not to have a mobile phone by your bedside holds a lot of truth. It isn't just scaremongers believing it can cause cancer, or more traditional souls who don't like these new-fangled gadgets. The blue light emitted from a smartphone can interfere with the natural hormones that help you sleep. In addition, the temptation mentally to look at something, respond to a message or even just think about doing that can prevent you from getting to sleep.

## Top tips

1 Don't use any backlit devices after a certain time in the evening if you are affected by this. You can use your sleep diary to work out what time works for you. I know my wife has a cut-off time of about 9 p.m. I don't seem to be affected by using a computer late into the evening. Work out what is right for you.

2 Keep all computers, tablets, smartphones out of the bedroom so that you are not tempted to use them when settling down to sleep or if you wake in the middle of the night. I hear people saying that they woke in the middle of the night and couldn't get back to sleep, so they got up and had a cup of tea and answered their emails. Spot the errors in this strategy!

# 28

# 'A little drink before bed helps me to sleep'

> Whoever drinks beer, he is quick to sleep; whoever sleeps long, does not sin; whoever does not sin, enters Heaven! Thus, let us drink beer!
>
> Martin Luther

I'm not sure how appropriate the Martin Luther quote is – sinning is not high on my plans for this book, and this chapter won't be discussing that – but in the first part, it does contain the phrase 'quick to sleep' when we have had a drink or two or three. Many of us know what this means. A night of drinking in a pub or restaurant, or at home with *Breaking Bad* on the television, quite often leads to falling asleep quickly. There is no doubt that the sedative effect of alcohol will make sleep come on faster than is normal without it, but the evidence points to the situation being much more complicated than this simple observation implies.

Society is so used to the idea of a drink in the evening, close to the time for bed, that we have borrowed a name for this practice: the nightcap. A nightcap was traditionally worn to bed in a bygone era as bedrooms were cold before central heating and reassured the wearer that it was time to sleep during the dark hours. Later the word came to be used instead to refer to an alcoholic drink had shortly before bedtime, so also has quite reassuring overtones. Surveys have shown that up to 15 per cent of people use alcohol regularly as a sleep aid.

## Alcohol affects the time taken to get to sleep

The effects of alcohol on sleep have interested science and medicine for a long time, the earliest recorded study being published in 1883, when Doctors Mönninghof and Piesbergen looked at how easy it was to wake someone who had been imbibing alcohol. Since then there have been many studies looking at ways alcohol affects sleep, and the impact of different amounts on the various stages of sleep.

A scientific paper published in 2013 summarized the evidence in a total of 20 studies from around the world, stating that regardless of how much alcohol we drink, we fall asleep more quickly after indulging in a tipple. The time in minutes it takes to get to sleep is known as sleep onset latency, which reduces with drinking alcohol before bedtime, regardless of the alcohol dose. Going to sleep more quickly is not the only effect: it seems that alcohol also increases the amount of time we spend in the deep-sleep stage. More time spent in deep sleep may seem like a good thing, as this is when the body lays down memories and adjusts your metabolism, but these apparently positive reasons for drinking alcohol also have knock-on effects on the whole night's sleep.

As you have possibly noticed when you have been drinking, across a whole night you are more likely to wake, perhaps to use the toilet or because of acid reflux or heartburn, causing sleep to be disrupted. Along with extra fluid swilling around your body, alcoholic drinks are diuretics, meaning they cause you to urinate more.

## There is less dreamtime with alcohol

There are also more subtle effects. If you drink heavily, which has been defined as more than four drinks in one session, you have less rapid eye movement (REM) sleep during the whole night. REM sleep is the part of the sleep cycle when you dream, and probably has a significant role on emotional states and memory. If you increase the amount of time in deep sleep, however, then something else has to give – usually, it seems, you get less of a dream-sleep stage.

After even just a few nights of regular drinking, the effect of falling asleep quickly wears off. Our bodies become tolerant of the alcohol. That is why you feel less effect from consuming it and so there may be the temptation to increase the dose, to increase the amount or strength, or both, of the drinks you have in order to replicate the original pleasurable experience.

## Alcohol makes you snore and possibly worse

Sleep apnoea is the name for when you are unable to breathe properly while asleep. There are two main types but the most common is known as obstructive sleep apnoea, in which your neck is unable to keep the breathing tube fully open and the lungs cannot take a sufficiently large breath. The result is that you are more likely to wake through the night.

If you do suffer from obstructive sleep apnoea, you must be careful, as alcohol is a relaxant and loosens your muscles. The relaxation feels good, and I know what effect this can have. Well, what I mean is that my wife knows: it makes me snore more. There can then be the knock-on effect of making the obstruction worse.

You must be very careful mixing alcohol with medications, and this includes sleep medications. There are some medications that, when combined with alcohol, cause harm, and this effect should be on the patient information leaflet. Note that the effectiveness of many other drugs will also be reduced when taking alcohol at the same time. Combining alcohol with pills that induce sleep, for example, can be dangerous and is generally warned against.

It is fine to have a drink now and then, but never use alcohol as a strategy for getting a better sleep. A recurring theme to the advice I give people, like Oscar Wilde, quoted earlier, is to use everything in moderation; including moderation. This is not saying you should give up drinking – that is against the ethos of restraint. For some people, such as those with dependency issues, giving up is clearly the correct thing to do, but not on the grounds that it hampers sleep. From the point of view of sleep, the 3-hour rule applies: finish the last sip 3 hours before you plan to go to bed. Before that, take it easy: one or two drinks within a day seems to be the healthiest approach.

The other, more obvious, issue of not staying up too late also applies. Plan the night out so that you can go to bed at close to your usual time. Then make sure you hydrate, and even then don't overdo the water drinking – remember it will fill your bladder; apologies for being blunt.

## Summary

Drinking alcohol certainly has a place in modern society, but it can be damaging for your sleep. You should not use it to induce sleep more rapidly, as tolerance may quickly develop. The sleep you get will be a lower quality than normal. You should also be aware of excessive snoring and the impact this may be having on your life.

## Top tips

1 Stop drinking alcohol 3 hours before bedtime.
2 Drink plenty of water, but not too much.
3 Don't use alcohol to induce sleep on a regular basis.

# 29

# 'A psychologist won't help me to sleep'

When you read the title of this chapter, you may agree with this statement and question how a psychologist could help anyone with sleep concerns. You might well think, 'I'm not crazy – why would a psychologist help?' A psychologist is a professional who studies human behaviour and mental processing. As a psychologist, Shane sees many patients with sleep concerns. Insomnia may be associated with other psychological conditions such as anxiety or depression or it may be a primary insomnia with no other underlying cause. Sleep affects mental health and mental health affects sleep. You can imagine it as a two-way street; difficulties with sleep are a symptom of difficulties with mood, letting you know something is amiss; and difficulties with sleep increase the likelihood of difficulties with mood.

This chapter will guide you through some psychological techniques that can help you sleep better. Of course, this is only a quick introduction, and if you feel you need more help, you should see a professional, either a psychologist or a general practitioner, to give you further help.

The sleep diary described in Chapter 1 is a reliable, validated tool for assessing your sleep. A 2-week sleep diary gives a good measure of sleep quality, in particular of how long it took to fall asleep, waking after sleep onset, total sleep time and sleep efficiency, which is the proportion of time spent in bed during which you are asleep.

## Psychological treatment of sleep concerns

There is a great deal of evidence that using psychological techniques to treat difficulties with sleep is as good as or better than using sleeping tablets. It has been proved that these techniques, unlike drugs, have long-term benefits with no risks. A commonly used technique is called cognitive behavioural therapy for insomnia (CBTi). This aims to change sleep habits as well as challenge beliefs about sleep that can worsen the situation. The technique uses both cognitive and behavioural interventions.

Let's start with the cognitive element. This is aimed at changing your misconceptions about sleep. You will probably recognize at this point that much of the book addresses exactly this: you need to know what normal sleep is so you can recognize whether or not yours is abnormal in some way. It is important to keep your expectations realistic and examine both internal and external causes of poor sleep. Cognitive therapy encourages you not to give sleep too much importance, not to catastrophize.

When you have difficulty sleeping there is a tendency to focus on this, which leads to a vicious circle, making you more anxious about sleeping, and then it becomes harder and harder to sleep. You will almost certainly have experienced this. Often people complain: 'I can't turn off my mind.' This is particularly common when there is a lot going on in your head, for example work, relationship or health worries. Other cognitive issues include false expectations, such as, 'I must sleep for 8 hours', or worrying about whether or not you are going to sleep. Trying to get to sleep in these situations inevitably increases the anxiety, and things get even worse. If these cognitive issues aren't addressed, they can turn into a long-term issue.

Cognitive therapy examines these beliefs and concerns and challenges them. The aim is to give you an alternative way of looking at sleep and more rational ways of viewing your difficulties. You may recognize that this is what this book is trying to do: who would have thought that by reading it you were actually having cognitive therapy?

There are simple cognitive techniques that you can try if you are having trouble falling asleep. Writing down a list of concerns, worries or tasks you have to do the following day, whatever the thoughts are that are filling your head, can be helpful. It is as if you are telling your brain to put these things aside while you sleep and you can pick them up again the following day. If you are still plagued by an active mind when trying to switch off, these thoughts can be stopped by repeating a random word like 'it' or 'the' in your head. These techniques take practice and are worth persisting with.

## Behavioural therapy

Whereas cognitive therapy focuses on the thoughts and beliefs you have about sleep, behavioural therapy is concerned with how your behaviours affect your sleep. Again you will see, when we look more at this, how much of this has been covered in the other chapters in this book.

One important part of behavioural therapy is called sleep hygiene. It's a rather clinical-sounding phrase but it looks at simple behaviours that can improve your sleep. The final chapter of this book, 'Sleep better', will cover this in detail so no more about it here. Other behavioural techniques Shane recommends that you may find helpful are stimulus-control therapy, muscle-relaxation training and sleep restriction. None of these techniques is going to change your sleep in one night. They all require practice, but experience has shown Shane that, if you do this, the results could be brilliant and may change your sleep.

Let us begin by looking at stimulus-control therapy. This sounds a bit scary but don't worry – it isn't. The aim of this therapy is to train you to associate the bedroom, and bed in particular, with sleep, and to establish a set sleep–wake programme. So how do you do this? Use your bedroom only for sleep and sex. It is really important not to watch television, work or eat in bed. You should also only go to bed when you feel sleepy; if you don't fall asleep within 15 minutes, then get up and leave the bedroom. Only come back to bed when you feel sleepy again. You can repeat this as often as necessary. This helps your mind to associate your bed and bedroom with sleeping and so trains your mind to get ready for sleep when you get into bed. The second aspect of this therapy is to get up at the same time every day, whether you have to get up for work or not, and try to avoid napping in the day. This way you help to set your internal clock, your circadian rhythm (see Chapter 15), so that you feel ready to sleep and ready to wake at the same time each day.

Another form of behavioural therapy is known as muscle relaxation training. Relaxation techniques are useful in treating anxiety, though they may help even if you are not anxious but find it hard to get to sleep. Progressive muscular relaxation has been shown to help promote sleep. In this technique you need to tense and relax your muscles in turn. Most people do this by starting at their feet and work up through the body. So start with the muscles in your feet; inhale and tense the foot muscles for a few seconds – this shouldn't be tense enough to cause pain or cramp in the muscles. Exhale and relax the feet. Stay relaxed for 10–15 seconds and then move on to the next muscle group: calves, thighs, buttocks and so on. You can either do both sides of the body at the same time or one side followed by the other – whatever works for you. While doing this, try to focus your thoughts on pleasant things, such as a beach, a favourite holiday spot, a picture you like, anything that helps you feel relaxed.

The final behavioural technique to look at is called sleep restriction. The name in itself sounds counterintuitive – you are trying to sleep better, not reduce your sleep – but don't worry, it does make sense. In this form of therapy you reduce the amount of time in bed in order to create a mild sleep deprivation, and then as your sleep efficiency improves (as you sleep for a greater proportion of the time you are in bed), you gradually lengthen the time you sleep for. Still sound confusing? Let's talk you through it.

You first need to use a sleep diary for 7–14 days to work out how much you are actually sleeping each night (see Chapter 1). You then need to restrict the time that you are in bed to the time that you actually slept each night during the period you kept the sleep diary. For example, if you spend 9 hours in bed each night but actually only sleep for 6 hours, you would only allow yourself 6 hours in bed each night. So if you normally go to bed at 11 p.m. but don't get to sleep until midnight, then wake for an hour in the night and get up at 7 p.m., you would need to go to bed at 1 a.m. and then still get up at 7 a.m. This stage will feel difficult. As you become more tired, you should find that you start to sleep for a lot longer during this 6-hour period. When you are sleeping for 90 per cent of the time you are in bed, then you can increase the time in bed by going to bed 15 minutes earlier and getting up at the same time. Continue increasing the time in 15-minute intervals until you find you are sleeping better and feeling refreshed in the morning.

## Summary

Cognitive behavioural therapy for insomnia has been proved to be an effective treatment. You probably thought at the start of this chapter that it sounded scary and difficult, but perhaps now you understand that it isn't scary, although it can be difficult. Changing thoughts and behaviours is not easy, which is why this book aims to give you some ideas about how you could improve your sleep.

## Top tips

1 Try one of the behavioural techniques described in this chapter and see if there is an effect on your sleep. Be realistic with yourself and don't expect changes overnight. You need to give any change a few weeks to see if there is an improvement in your sleep.
2 Look through the myths covered in this book and find the ones that apply most to you. Try implementing the tips in that chapter and making them part of your daily life. Just by doing that you are engaging with cognitive behavioural therapy.

# 30

# 'If I slept less I could get more done'

A single day is a finite period of time. There are 24 hours, no more. It makes sense, then, that if you reduce the time you spend doing one thing, you will increase the time available for other things. That's logical. Therefore if you could reduce the amount of time spent sleeping, you could increase the time you have for work or fun.

There are many ways in which you could try to reduce time spent asleep, but would it help?

## How do you spend your time?

I read about a woman who worked really hard to change her sleep schedule. She made an extra 2–3 hours available each day, which now could be used for waking activities. Then the challenge became: what was she to do with this time? She ended up taking up knitting, making jumpers and hats. This, presumably, is productive for some, but it was clear from the tone that she was not impressed.

So let's start by asking what you get done in an hour, a day, a week, a year. Have you given this any thought? I hear from many people that they 'don't have enough time', often in relation to doing something specific. I really don't ever feel, if I am being truthful with myself, that I have too little time. The reality is that I could make time, but I don't want to. It may be something I am not keen on or don't have sufficient motivation to achieve. So my lack of time is really all about my lack of motivation or will to carry out that thing.

## Spending extra time at work?

Let's think about doing more work, as this seems to be one motivation for sleeping less. Your time working only takes a proportion of your hours awake. If you are concerned that you need to increase the amount of work you do, then rather than think about the increased amount of time you could spend working, why not increase the amount of work you do in a similar amount of time? This will be by increasing productivity.

Interestingly, some employers are now working on this, acknowledging that you must get sufficient sleep in order for you to have more quality time at work. Understandably the employers want more work for each pound, euro or dollar. To give just one example, members of staff at a forward-thinking insurance firm can claim £240 ($300) each year by declaring their sleep. When they have slept at least 7 hours per night, they are rewarded. Now that may not seem fair for people who struggle with their sleep, but a further motivation may help, and 25,000 members of staff signed up for it.

This obviously relies on trust, which is also a good attitude to have. You empower your members of staff, trusting them to do the right thing and speak the truth. There are many wins, both for the employer and the employees.

## Spend more time in leisure?

Finally, something that won't be dwelt on here is having more leisure time. Because of the way society is structured, many hours during the night are not set up, not convenient for pursuing leisure activities. Most happen in the normal daytime hours or early evening. If you have more time, most other people do not. So what are you to do? One study showed that the boredom from this extra time can lead to filling these hours with eating. The natural consequence of this extra time, and extra food, is extra weight. This is discussed more in Chapter 2.

## Summary

There are ways you can increase your time awake, but you should be careful. You need to consider what you want to achieve with more time. Do you want to work? Or have some leisure activity? These may be best pursued during normal waking hours, and the extra time will then be filled with less productive pastimes. There is an adage: 'Be careful what you wish for.'

## Top tips

1 Think about what you do in a day and if more time will really help.
2 Consider increases in productivity. Use modern technology to best effect.
3 Sign up, where you can, for rewards for good sleep.

# 31

# 'I can catch up on my sleep any time'

We humans have organized our lives in a curious way. However this came about, we seem, in westernized society at least, to have split a repeating time frame that we call a week into two distinct phases: 5 weekdays and 2 days of weekend. This can have profound and significant impacts on our health, well-being and life.

## Weekday and weekend days are treated differently

It is fairly traditional for many people to work for the 5 weekdays and then not over the weekend, although this distinction is breaking up, with the changes in retail and service sectors.

Another consequence of this distinction between weekdays and weekends is the interesting concept of the weekday vegetarian. I came across this in Taiwan, a country where a large proportion of the population are Buddhist and therefore try to avoid eating animals. Vegetarianism can be a difficult choice for many people, though, so some choose to take a more flexible approach, sometimes called a flexitarian diet. This has led them to avoid eating meat on weekdays but to eat it at the weekend.

What is the point of talking about this? It is because many people in the West apply this approach to their sleep lives. During the weekdays you can lose sleep for many different reasons. You may have to get up earlier than your body wants to, as your alarm goes off and you must drag yourself out of bed and off to work. Your job may need you to work late into the evening, or you may have a social life that leads to late nights, which reduce the window of time for you to sleep. This leads to a sleep debt, which is the name for the effect of not getting enough sleep.

Everybody has a different level at which a debt will be accrued, and this will lead to cognitive effects, such as irritability, poor judgement and increased reaction times. All these will be in some way proportionate to the amount of sleep debt accrued, but within the scientific community, there is no generally agreed definition of when a sleep debt is started, nor a way to quantify the effects objectively.

The effects may be seen in different ways. You may feel very sluggish when you wake, relying on the alarm clock, and this feeling may last a number of hours. You may feel sleepy in meetings, when driving or on a train. After work you may fall asleep on the sofa, at the meal table or while watching television.

## Repaying your sleep debt

So what do you do when you are in sleep debt? It has become a common approach to feel that the weekend is the time that allows you to catch up on your sleep. This may be through trying to go to bed earlier that you do normally on a weekday, although this may not work because your body fights attempts to sleep earlier than what it considers 'normal'. Another approach, and probably the most common, is to sleep in later in the morning. This will help to relieve some of the debt; help to pay it back.

Some people suggest that you can work out your sleep debt by adding up the number of hours you feel you have lost. This may be over the past few days or even weeks. It does rely on your knowing what your normal sleeping hours should be (avoiding the 8-hour trap – see Chapter 1), which in turn requires that you keep some sort of sleep diary (Chapter 1 again). Then, once your debt is calculated as a number of hours, you sleep that on top of your normal sleep time.

This sounds very complex, fraught with uncertainty, despite offering you some sort of reassurance that the use of numbers will make it more 'scientific' or a 'better' approach. It doesn't seem a useful method. Rather, you should rely on how you feel – if you feel you are as good as you can be. Because we are all different, this is a helpful definition of health: if, within your physical, mental and emotional bounds, you are as good as you can be, then you could describe yourself as healthy.

There are two important points to make about this repayment approach. The first is that the repayment may allow you to feel better – to restore your mental powers to where they were before the debt was accrued. The other, more invisible effects, particularly on your metabolism, cannot be recovered, however. It is too late for you to think you can somehow repair any metabolic damage done during the sleepiness phase.

The second point is the possible consequence that your body, after 2 days of sleeping in late in the morning, may then really struggle to get back on track on the weekday. You may not feel sleepy on the Sunday night, past your normal weekday bedtime, which will have a knock-on effect on Monday morning.

## Summary

There are any number of different reasons for sleep being disturbed. One of these is the weekend and weekday differences, which may lead to an accrual of a sleep debt. This is a notional number of hours of sleep you owe your body. It has become a fairly trendy notion, which suggests you can somehow repay this debt and, just like a financial debt, it can be paid off with no further consequences. This is not correct. You may recover some of the immediately lost functions, such as reaction times and thinking power, but there are other effects that cannot be recovered, particularly in relation to your metabolic health.

## Top tips

1  Try not to accrue a sleep debt.
2  If you do, consider organizing a pretty swift repayment.
3  Try to manage your sleep in a fairly consistent fashion, so you do not have a weekday accrual of sleep debt.

# 32

# 'I'm too busy to have breakfast'

As Virginia Woolf said, sleeping well usually does mean you need to eat well, but many people are 'too busy' to have breakfast. Yes, breakfast does take a few minutes. My wife and I eat muesli every morning, which we make the night before – but, still, 10 minutes are 'wasted'. Your parents may have said that breakfast is the most important meal of the day; I know mine did. More recently, in opposition to this, you may have heard people say that they don't have time to squeeze it in and they are trying to lose weight. You may have said it yourself.

Going without breakfast is a common practice among many people in our society. In fact, a study at the University of Edinburgh in 2010 found that more than 50 per cent of 15-year-old girls were missing breakfast every morning. This is a worrying figure, as I would imagine that if you are regularly skipping breakfast as a teenager, this will become a habit that stays with you for the rest of your life.

There are two reasons breakfast is very important for your sleep. Using time and wanting to lose weight as excuses not to eat breakfast is plain wrong, and the reasons for this are your metabolism and your circadian rhythm. If you are struggling with your sleep and feel the need to have every last moment in warm slumber, it can be difficult to tell yourself to get up and eat. It's not intuitive; nevertheless it is what you should strive to do.

## Metabolism is primed by breakfast

Rather than go into loads of detail on how hormones and your biochemistry operate, especially glucose and insulin, the reality is that we seem able to operate best when we break our fast in the morning. If we start our day without eating, our body must deal with energy use, moving our muscles, setting our bodies going to react to whatever comes our way. Our cortisol levels have an impact on our sleep, and the level of this hormone in our bloodstream rises first thing in the morning, getting us up and started. As the day drags on, these levels drop until tiredness overcomes us.

This hormone does more than regulate energy levels and sleep, though. When your body uses up glucose for doing things, such as moving and thinking, your blood glucose drops. This leads to your producing more cortisol, allowing glucose to flood into your veins and arteries. This is done by your adrenal cortex, lying above your kidneys, which monitors your cortisol all the time, giving you bursts of hormones for glucose to be used when you need it.

Your overnight fast is usually in the region of 12–14 hours since your last meal, which would normally be your evening meal, so long as you haven't also snacked later. If you can replenish your blood glucose by eating food first thing in the morning, you won't need to produce cortisol. You are giving your glands some love with a boost of sugar and no need to resort to plan B, which is that having no breakfast results in your adrenal cortex producing cortisol to release the glucose you need.

This amount of cortisol is greater than you need, however, which then also sets a level higher throughout the day, which will also carry on into the night. Your job is to try to keep cortisol to a lower, more appropriate level in the day, ready for the night. High cortisol will stop you from relaxing and gaining sleep time. Other things that can also contribute to this are stress, caffeine and skipping other meals.

The breakfast will also give your body a better, more regulated, eating pattern, which allows your body to regulate glucose better. Skipping any meal can lead to craving sweet things.

## Eating plays an important role in your body rhythms

Your body is governed by its own internal clock, which we know as the circadian rhythm (see Chapters 15 and 34). These rhythms are controlled by our using external cues continually to check and modify where we are in the day and in the night. This process of using these cues is known as entrainment, and we use many different cues. These include light and dark, temperature and, importantly, our meals.

Eating at the correct time tells our body either to wind down or to wake up. Breaking our fast is one of the cues for our body to get going; in fact it has been suggested that meals are even more important than sunlight in this process. As said above, you must also stop eating – that is, you must start fasting – the day before, preferably 12 hours or more before you are to wake up. Failure to stop eating and start fasting, in other words snacking, can lead to unwanted weight gain.

## Dealing with the morning craziness

Imagine someone told you that you could eat more food without gaining weight. Most people who enjoy their food would jump at the chance. Well, a study in 2008 of 6,764 men and women at Addenbrooke's Hospital, Cambridge, found that people who ate the most for breakfast put on the least amount of weight over the years that the study ran, even though they typically ate the most food in total through the day. Many studies, in both adults and children, have shown that people who eat breakfast tend to weigh less than those who don't. A study of more than 2,000 girls aged 9–19 found that eating breakfast regularly was associated with fewer issues regarding weight. The girls who ate breakfast infrequently were 13 per cent more likely to be overweight than those who ate breakfast regularly. I know my scientist colleagues will be shouting that this may just be due to bias in the science, but I see no reason why this research should be ignored.

I discovered Bircher muesli while on holiday a few years ago in Australia; funny how travelling to another country introduces you to new ideas. This changed my breakfast eating habits and I now eat it every day. It is very simple to make, only requiring you to put some oats and milk into a bowl and leave for 8 hours or more. Do this in the evening and leave it in the fridge overnight, and there is breakfast waiting for you when you get up in the morning. I add dried fruits, nuts and seeds, and play around with the mix in the interests of variety.

A recent trend is the production of cereal bars and breakfast biscuits. These are marketed for eating on the go by those too busy to sit down and have breakfast, but are they a good option? When their nutritional content is analysed they are generally found to have a high sugar content; in fact most of these breakfast bars have more sugar than many normal biscuits. Unfortunately, eating a breakfast high in sugar causes your sugar level to peak and then rapidly drop; this drop in sugar level makes you crave more sugar, which is a common cause of snacking later in the morning.

However, most do contain whole grains, which are beneficial when eaten for breakfast. An additional negative aspect to such an on-the-go breakfast is that it encourages people to eat mindlessly, which is a behaviour commonly associated with weight gain. My opinion is that it is much better to take time to sit down and eat breakfast, and to make sensible choices about what to eat. However, as we have seen, eating breakfast in itself is beneficial, and it may be that eating anything is better than eating nothing.

## Summary

Skipping breakfast is a fairly common strategy for many people, based on the perceived reduction in calories and need to save time. It is true that some people have no wish to eat, but this can be a learnt behaviour over time. Those who eat breakfast seem to start their metabolic day in a better way than those who don't. It may also have a good impact on your body's natural rhythm, setting your day up for the night ahead.

## Top tips

1  Eat breakfast.
2  Eat breakfast.

# 33

# 'Never go to sleep on an argument'

My wife's uncle is a lovely man. He very graciously agreed to speak at our wedding, and read a poem by Wilferd Peterson that said we should never go to sleep angry with our partner. It seems like common advice, and must be a good thing for a marriage, but does it have an impact on your sleep? The whole idea seems obvious. You may have experienced negative feelings while you lie in bed, trying to get to sleep. These feelings can magnify and dominate your mind, when you should be trying to stop thinking. A thinking mind struggles to fall asleep.

A study of over 600 people in the USA has shown that those who feel most valued by their partner have a better quality of sleep. They experience lower anxiety, which helps them to relax and achieve deep sleep. The actual bit about 'never going to sleep angry', however, is about the way it affects your marriage and I can safely say that, in my experience, this is so true. Speaking clearly and honestly about feelings is the best way to deal with the bumps in the road. These are found in every marriage or relationship, and you need to put in the effort to resolve them.

There doesn't seem to have been a study looking at whether or not the resolution of arguments before sleep makes for a better marriage. Seems like a good project – I'll start writing a grant application . . .

## Summary

Evidence supports the view that having a good relationship helps sleep. Whether or not the resolution of arguments before sleep is the best approach, it does seem worth a try.

## Top tip

1 Your sleep may be, in part, governed by having a good relationship. You may need to work on your life with your partner to help your sleep.

# 34

# 'I won't come to any harm from not sleeping'

In a play written by the famous author E. M. Forster called *The Machine Stops*, the end of the world is brought on when the beds fail to appear. The collapse of humanity might seem a little extreme, although there are some real examples of sleepiness leading to terrible accidents, such as the Chernobyl nuclear explosion and the Exxon Valdez oil spill disaster. We will start with a very sad story about a real person. In 1985 a paper was published that told us about a 53-year-old man who attended a hospital in Bologna in Italy. This beautiful city, lined with porticos, founded one of the first universities in the world. The city's beauty was not important to this man as he struggled to live with a terrible disease. This disease is now known as fatal familial insomnia, whereby the person cannot achieve any restful sleep. Doctors tried to use anaesthetics and drugs but these did not work, as he still continued to fail to sleep. Over the course of a few months his condition got worse. After 9 months, he died.

This dramatic event is clear evidence that we cannot survive without sleep. Since then, 40 families have been found to have this very rare genetic disorder and sadly no progress has been made to help these poor people.

We are taught at school that humans need oxygen, water and food to survive. It is also taken for granted that we need shelter to protect us from temperature changes. Despite knowing about this fatal disease, we are not taught that sleep is also essential; and we need it every night. We do intuitively understand, however, the central role that sleep plays in our lives.

## What happens if I don't sleep?

In 1964 a young man, 17 years old, took part in a school experiment. Randy Gardner stayed awake for over 11 days, attended by an expert in sleep, Dr William Dement, and a US Navy scientific researcher, Lieutenant Commander John J. Ross, who monitored his health. Even after this extreme behaviour he did not have any lasting physical or mental effects. However, he wasn't able to behave normally during the period when he was deprived of sleep; his brain had lost all its power to function normally. After only a few days of not sleeping, for example, he was unable to carry out simple mental arithmetic.

You will probably be able to describe how you feel when you do not get enough sleep. I know that when my children woke my wife and me during the night, I felt empty. My body was whole but my mind was absent.

Rest assured that, unless you suffer from the insomnia disorder described above, there has not been a single case of someone actually dying from sleep deprivation directly. There are large numbers of issues that come from not sleeping, however. Many of these are hidden, beyond our straightforward feelings of tiredness and fatigue.

Apart from these feelings of lethargy, sleep deprivation can lead to a lack of motivation, moodiness and irritability. Depending on the amount and type of your work and play, there can be reduction in creativity and problem-solving skills, poorer ability to cope with stress, lack of concentration and poor memory. In addition to these mental symptoms, which we can all recognize, research has recently identified that there may also be physical symptoms, such as reduced immunity, a gain in weight and longer-term health issues, such as diabetes and heart-related conditions.

In fact sleep deprivation can affect you just as much as being drunk. There have been some estimates of this effect, which is subject to all sorts of variation, such as caffeine intake and sleep debt. It seems that if you were to stay awake for 21 hours, your ability to drive is similar to having drunk up to the legal limit of alcohol intake for driving in the UK, which is 0.08 per cent (80 milligrams of alcohol in 100 millilitres of blood).

## Sleep debt can build up

Being unable to sleep leads to the build-up of sleep debt (see Chapter 31). This debt can cause you to have increased anxiety, shorter attention span, a reduction in memory and low mood. You may have lower ability to perform difficult thought processes: calculations, planning and strategic decision-making.

Unfortunately the sleep debt makes it sound as though it is something we can easily keep track of, as we do our personal bank finances, but there is not a number, a figure in hours, that we owe ourselves. This also makes it very difficult to make any sort of recommendation to guide people on their sleeping. Adding to this confusion, there is no agreement of what debt is 'allowable' – at what point does your body call in the bailiffs? If you have realized you have a debt, you can try to repay your sleep debt, which will generally be reversed, but it is not as straightforward as that. Sleeping isn't something you can do whenever you want, as you probably know. Sleep comes on when your mind wants to sleep.

Much of this is to do with what is called your circadian rhythm, where your body has a 24-hour routine based on cues from all around you (see also Chapter 15). These cues include light and dark, mealtimes, exercise and social activity. You've probably had the experience of feeling tired but your body refusing to sleep. Much of this is because of your circadian rhythm. This effect goes a little further, too: your circadian rhythm will tend to wake you at your 'usual' wake-up time. This may mean it is difficult to repay your sleep debt fully.

There are no rules about when you reach the point of maximum sleepiness. My wife, who trained to be a doctor in the 1990s, would frequently remain awake for 36 hours. She was, throughout this time, in charge of life-and-death situations, and people's lives depended on her correct decision-making under pressure.

Many scientific research studies show that the amount of time you sleep may have an impact on how long you live. The slightly tricky issue comes when you look at some of the detail. It is what we call a U-shaped curve, where at a low amount of sleep the risk of death is higher (the left of the letter U), reducing in the middle of the U with sleep of 6–9 hours per night.

Then a little more surprisingly, on the right-hand side of the letter U there is an increase in risk of death with high levels of sleep – over 9 hours per night. The jury remains out on whether this is a cause of death or just a side effect of some other thing that leads to death. The longer time sleeping is a particularly challenging part, where some suggestions are that it is due to fatigue from an underlying disease, such as cancer, or as a symptom of depression.

## Summary

it is clearly not good to either not sleep or sleep too much. There are serious diseases that may be caused by too little sleep and it may even have an impact on your safety. Sleep debt may build up, and you need to think carefully about this, but also pay attention to sleeping too much.

## Top tips

1 Look at the amount of time you spend asleep, using the sleep diary in Chapter 1.
2 Pay attention to too little sleep, and what this means to your sleep debt.
3 Also be careful of excessive sleep, as this may indicate other things such as psychological issues (see Chapter 29) or sleep apnoea (see Chapter 35).

# 35

# 'Snoring means I'm sleeping well'

This is an interesting myth, though it's unclear where it comes from or how anybody thought it was real. The comical element sometimes attached to our perceptions of snoring masks how serious it can be. Snoring starts when there is too much relaxation of the airway muscles and they vibrate together. When we breathe while sleeping, the air moves these muscles and a sound like a chainsaw can be the result. It happens to most of us at some time, but it can impede good sleep, and if you are sleeping next to a snorer, then definitely it is going to have an impact on you.

You must be careful if you are a snorer, too. Snoring may indicate that you have sleep apnoea, which can be a serious disorder that occurs during sleep when your breathing repeatedly stops. The word 'apnoea' literally means 'without breath', and is defined as cessation of breathing for 10 seconds or longer. You are in no immediate danger – your body is amazing, and you wake yourself gently to start breathing again. You may do this many, many times in a single night, however, and so your brain is unable to fall into the most restorative deep sleep because it is busy regaining control over your breathing.

You may have been told that you are a snorer, and your bed partner may remark that he or she thinks you have stopped breathing. You may also wake feeling as though you are struggling with your breathing, or even feel that you are choking. These overnight activities may mean you are tired during the day, with a feeling of grogginess. This can seem confusing because you may think you slept for an appropriate length of time, but your body is not fully refreshed because you repeatedly woke up.

Cognitive deficits – for example in visual memory, speed tasks, short-term memory, long-term memory, visuo-spatial performance – are also a consequence. Sleep apnoea is related to depression, sleepiness and drowsiness. It is also related to metabolic disorders, high blood pressure and kidney disease.

## Ways to reduce snoring

Snoring, and therefore possibly sleep apnoea, is more likely to occur in those who are overweight and also more generally in men. The best we can do to manage snoring is to prevent its likelihood in the first place. This can be done by weight loss, using positional therapy to avoid lying face upwards when sleeping, and of course avoiding alcohol. Many ways of reducing snoring have been tried – getting the snorer to sleep on his side or front rather than on his back may work.

There are medical interventions to reduce snoring, the main one being a device known as a CPAP – an abbreviation for continuous positive airway pressure. This delivers mild air pressure to your lungs through your mouth or nose, which will reduce the frequency and intensity of snoring and improve sleep quality for those who snore and those who sleep next to them. Improvements to quality-of-life measures are also more likely. These devices continue to be improved, but people using them will experience some side effects, which include a feeling of claustrophobia from the mask, or nasal congestion.

## Summary

Snoring should not be ignored. It can have serious consequences for the quality of your life. There are ways to treat it. The most important consideration is the weight of the person who snores.

## Top tips

1 Don't ignore your snoring. If you are told you snore, take it seriously. Consider what to do about it.
2 If you are concerned about tiredness, and particularly if you have been told that you snore, consider going to see your general practitioner to discuss options.
3 Losing weight will help to reduce the amount and frequency of snoring.

# 36

# 'A banana before bed
helps me to sleep'

My mother-in-law told me some years ago that eating a banana before bed helps promote a good night's sleep. Knowing that she is banana obsessed and had previously told me that bananas are good for cleaning shoes and healing sore bottoms, I was more than a little sceptical. I decided to look into it further and see if there was any evidence that this myth was true.

I found several promising articles saying bananas contain potassium and magnesium, which help muscles relax. They also contain an amino acid called tryptophan, which is converted into serotonin, a chemical that your body uses to help you relax, and melatonin, a chemical that helps promote sleepiness. It was looking as though there was some truth in this old wives' tale. However, I was unable to find any scientific evidence that confirmed bananas truly help you sleep better. It is thought that levels of tryptophan in bananas are not high enough to have any real effect on sleep.

## Other food products may help you sleep

You have probably heard that a milky drink before bed will help you sleep, an often-quoted idea long used to market a well-known malted milk drink in the UK. The rationale behind this is, once again, that dairy products contain tryptophan, but, as with bananas, it is thought there isn't enough in them for it to be effective. Other foods high in tryptophan include nuts and seeds, honey and eggs.

Foods that logically should improve sleep are those that are naturally high in melatonin, and one of these that has been studied is tart Montmorency cherries. A study in 2012 randomized 20 participants to 7 days of placebo – as in a suitable replacement, but not the same product – or tart cherry juice concentrate. Those who had the cherry juice had higher urinary melatonin levels and their sleep was longer and of better quality than those who had the placebo. Perhaps if other foods were studied, we might find that they too do truly improve sleep.

## Some foods can make your sleep worse

So can what you eat affect your sleep? Researchers in a study carried out in New York looked at the impact of diet on sleep. They recruited 26 normal-weight adults with no trouble sleeping. Their sleep was monitored each night in a sleep lab. For the first 4 days of the study, they were all given a controlled diet and, on the final day, were free to eat as they chose. The amount of sleep each participant had didn't vary during the days on the controlled diet and the final day, but the sleep quality was worse on the final night – all took longer to get to sleep and slept worse. Eating more saturated fat caused worse sleep, and more sugar and other carbohydrates resulted in more waking during the night. Now this was only a small study and many other factors may have been involved other than the diet, but it provides some evidence that diet can have an impact on sleep quality.

You almost certainly know the uncomfortable feeling of eating a large meal before going to bed. The digestive system slows down when you sleep, meaning you feel overly full for longer. In addition, a full stomach can lead to acid reflux symptoms, and lying flat makes this more uncomfortable. To prevent this, it is generally best to eat your evening meal a few hours before going to bed. Indeed, I heard from Arabic colleagues the saying that you should eat like a poor person at night, otherwise you will have nightmares.

However, it is also difficult to fall asleep if you are feeling hungry, so a small snack before bed may be beneficial. Perhaps this is where bananas and milk come in – it would seem sensible to choose foods that help to promote sleep when choosing an evening snack. Don't forget to beware of caffeine before bed; coffee before bed is obviously not a good choice but chocolate, cocoa, cola and tea also contain caffeine.

## Summary

Food may affect how much sleep you get and how good it is. Bananas and milk products have been suggested to help you get to sleep, but there is no clear reason why this might be. Some foods seem definitely to spoil your sleep and are best avoided.

## Top tips

1 If you find falling asleep difficult, consider a light food, maybe a banana or better still a milky drink.
2 If you struggle with your sleep, think about what you eat and when. Are large, oily fatty meals sitting on your stomach? Think about eating earlier and consider what you are eating.

# 37

# 'The older I get, the more sleep I need'

I really like the saying 'At some point you stop growing up and start growing older.' This feels a nice way to look at the trajectory of your life, that change happens with time. It is common that, with increasing age, changes happen to your sleep.

At the beginning of life, babies sleep a great deal, spending up to three-quarters of their day asleep, shutting their eyes when they want and, to some extent, where they want. Society is also starting to recognize that although teenagers seem to sleep too much, it is their job; a natural and important part of their development includes changes to their sleep schedule.

Mixed in with this patchwork of acceptance and criticism, our society commonly tends to view older people as not only well-loved members of the family but also as people who fall asleep in their armchairs after a meal. I have fond memories of watching my Grandad be woken up by my Grandmother after Christmas dinner: 'Wake up, Den.'

## Evidence tells us that older people sleep less

So we may tend to think that older people sleep more and need more sleep to function normally. The evidence, though, does not support this.

Surveys report that older people sleep less over the course of a full day than younger people. In data from a UK study called Understanding Society, we can see that sleep varies considerably with age. As people reach their twenties, they reduce their sleep time from teenage years to what we recognize as a more standard amount of time asleep, 7–9 hours. This carries on reducing until around the age of 50, when there is an increase again.

Then by the time people are in their seventies, on average they're generally sleeping 45 minutes less than they did when in their twenties. Remember that this is an average, a number used by scientists, and it doesn't mean it will happen in your case; it is just more likely it will. The least time spent asleep occurs at the oldest ages in women. However, in men the reported amount of sleep remains just above 7 hours per night. People also report more insomnia as they age. Nearly half of all people over 65 report at least one concern they have with their sleep.

When I ask people of different ages to come to my sleep laboratory and have their brain activity measured while they sleep, an interesting pattern emerges. Young people, those in their teens and twenties, have very clear deep sleep: the brain waves demonstrate powerful and long-lasting deep sleep. Speaking from personal experience, when you have the honour to reach your mid-forties, deep sleep has dramatically reduced, as my colleagues showed when I spent the night in my sleep laboratory all wired up.

## Changes in your life have an impact on sleep

There are many reasons why sleep changes as you get older. This may be due to the development of chronic conditions and medications that interfere with good sleep, or the psychology of ageing and the differences in life brought about by changes in mobility and occupation. Or it may simply be that we need less sleep as we age.

There are also changes in people's lives that have a big impact on the amount of sleep they can have. People with babies and young children have less sleep – often less than they want. The menopause in women can also have a dramatic effect on the amount of sleep it is possible to have. These phases shouldn't last for ever and people usually return to their favoured patterns.

There may be neurological reasons, stuff that happens in your brain and nervous system as you age, which mean that your sleep is different from how you would like it to be. A recent scientific study found a cluster of cells, called the ventrolateral preoptic nucleus, that regulate sleep patterns and die off as we get older. The researchers went on further to say that the elderly do sleep but do not feel rested, partly because of this regulation system being lost. In fact, they described it as a sort of chronic insomnia state that older people in our society may experience.

## Different health-related and other difficulties come with age and affect sleep

Our weight has a big impact on how we sleep, particularly how well we breathe. Most people's weight changes as they age. Snoring is often caused by extra weight around the neck, and can be a major cause of sleep disruption. Reports from the USA state that over a quarter of adults have disrupted sleep due to snoring and excess weight.

Other sleep disorders can become more prevalent as you get older. An example of this is restless legs syndrome, where you have an irresistible urge to move your limbs, usually your legs. This may happen at any point during the day but gets worse as the night draws in. These feelings of tingling and restlessness can interfere with getting to sleep, as you want to get up and walk around. There also seems to be some association between this and what is known as periodic limb movement disorder, which is where your legs or arms move involuntarily, usually while you are asleep. This also occurs more as you get older.

As we age there is also an increase in the likelihood that we will suffer from chronic conditions that are not directly a disorder of sleep but indirectly have a large impact. Disorders that cause pain, such as arthritis, will make it hard to get to sleep and to maintain sleep all night. There are many other chronic conditions that we can treat and survive, but they still affect our sleep. For example, a survivor of cancer often struggles with sleep. In addition, for various disorders, the treatment that can help us live longer and happier lives can also affect our sleep.

Increasing levels of worry and stress may be due to work issues, family difficulties and a fear of death. People with Alzheimer's disease seem to lose more rapidly the brain cells that regulate sleep. We don't understand how this process operates, but it affects those with the disease, their families and their carers. Losing a loved one, particularly a spouse, can leave you feeling isolated and lonely. This often leads to trouble sleeping and depression. Surveys show that 75 per cent of recent widows have a hard time sleeping a month after the death of their spouse. One year later, 50 per cent report that their sleep difficulties still have not gone away.

Finally, there is the practical issue of needing the bathroom. Most people over the age of 65 get up at least once during the night. These disruptions have different impacts on different people.

## Summary

Sleep varies as you get older. You probably will not sleep as much as when you were a baby or a teenager, but after retirement you may sleep more than when you went to work. Some of these changes are also dependent on different factors, including the development of chronic disorders, such as Alzheimer's disease, changes in weight and hormone balance. In addition, there is evidence that cell death in your brain may play a role in losing control of your sleep schedule.

## Top tips

1 If you are lucky enough to get older, then embrace your sleep patterns; enjoy any changes, either more time awake or more time to sleep.
2 Consider seeking help for long-term diseases and disorders that may be having an impact on your sleep.
3 Consider your weight, particularly in relation to sleep apnoea.

# 38

# 'My laptop takes up little room in my bedroom'

I am not a Luddite; I embrace new technology; I am an early adopter. Among my friends, I was one of the first to get an iPod, causing great hilarity, but I am afraid I am going to have a moan about technology now. Well, not exactly technology but when and where it is used.

I find it slightly depressing how people use laptops in their bedrooms. They are amazing pieces of technology; indeed, most of this book was written on one. The portability allows their use in the café, in the kitchen, at work or on the train. Your bedroom, though. is for two things: sleeping and sex. You don't need a laptop for either of these. Perhaps you have no other room in which to work, but if there is any way you can work elsewhere, you should try to do so. The trouble with laptops is the blue light, sounds and stimulation that accompany using the screen to work or play games.

Your body needs quiet calmness in preparation for sleeping, and a laptop offers so many opportunities to get your mind working. You may want to have intimate, personal conversation with your bed partner, or mindful reflection on the decisions of the day. Again a laptop will interrupt this: it is so tempting.

There is no need, for most people, to have immediate access in bed to email, Facebook, Twitter, any social media. Nothing will change – really, nothing will change. You may even end up sending messages you wouldn't have done were you wide awake, firing on all cylinders. There is no need to experience the emotional roller-coaster that can come with social media.

Ultimately all the rooms in your house should serve a purpose. You should decide what these are and stick to that (see Chapter 40). Unfortunately some companies now market a laptop bed table, allowing you to sit on your bed and use your screen.

These guidelines are particularly important for teenagers, as their sleep is so important to their well-being. A study in Norway of 100,000 children found that they used electronic devices extensively in their bedrooms at bedtime. This use led to it taking longer for them to fall asleep and less time asleep, many having fewer than 6 hours per night.

## Summary

There is a strong temptation to take your laptop, or any similar device, to bed to work and to use the internet. Switching off, disconnecting, can induce distress: are you missing something? You should try to avoid this behaviour, use your bedroom for sleep and sex, and try not to relate to it as a place of work. Calming, gentle reading or talking will allow your body to understand where you are in your daily rhythm.

## Top tips

1  Avoid using your laptop in, or even taking it to, to your bedroom.
2  Define the use for each of your rooms, and stick to those uses.
3  Keep your bedroom free from electronics and sources of blue light.

# 39

# 'I can just take a tablet to help me with my sleep'

Every year in England, more than 10 million prescriptions for sleeping pills are given out by doctors. This would appear, on the face of it, to be a very simple solution for anyone who has trouble getting off to sleep. Sleeping tablets reduce the length of time taken to fall asleep and increase the amount of time spent sleeping. So why is this not the answer to all sleep issues? Sadly, while in the short term they can work, long-term use of sleeping tablets is not advisable.

Current guidelines in the UK advise doctors that sleeping tablets should be prescribed at the lowest dose possible for the shortest time possible, and only if all other solutions are inappropriate or ineffective. Why is this?

Let's begin by looking at what drugs are used to aid sleep. Chloral hydrate, developed in 1832, is thought to be the earliest drug clinically used for insomnia. Unfortunately, the dose needed to induce sleep was not much less than the lethal dose, so it was not uncommon to die from an overdose. Chloral hydrate was also used in the original 'Mickey Finn', slipped into the drink of an unsuspecting person who would then be robbed while incapacitated.

Barbiturates were then discovered and widely used in the early twentieth century as sleeping aids. These are addictive drugs, however, and can also be lethal in overdose. Elvis Presley, Marilyn Monroe and Jim Morrison each died from an overdose of sleeping pills. Benzodiazepines have been the drug of choice since the 1960s, as these have lower abuse potential and are less risky in overdose. They were developed and widely used for anxiety and panic attacks, but they also helped people sleep. As they were so much safer than barbiturates, doctors began prescribing them for insomnia. Valium, a benzodiazepine, was the most commonly prescribed drug in the USA between 1969 and 1982. Their use in insomnia has declined with the introduction in the 1990s of the 'z-drugs', which are similar to benzodiazepines but with quicker onset of action, less 'hangover' the following day and fewer side effects. These benefits over benzodiazepines have been questioned since their introduction, but nevertheless today these are the dominant prescription sleeping tablets. During the 12-month period from December 2011 to November 2012, over 6 million prescriptions for z-drugs were dispensed in England.

A newer tablet for insomnia has become available in the UK in the last few years. Melatonin can now be prescribed for adults with insomnia over the age of 55. Melatonin is a naturally occurring hormone in our bodies that causes sleepiness. Again this is recommended for short-term use only, and similar to other sleeping tablets it can cause drowsiness the following morning. It can also cause headaches, joint pains and cold-like symptoms.

In addition to these prescription sleeping tablets there are also some sleeping aids that can be bought over the counter. You have probably heard of Nytol, and there are other similar tablets. These generally contain an antihistamine, which can cause drowsiness. They are generally not recommended, as it isn't clear how effective they actually are and obviously they can cause side effects or interact with any other medications you take.

## Prescribed drugs have unintended consequences

So it seems we now have drugs for insomnia that do work and do appear to be safe if taken as prescribed. So, once again, why is this not the answer to all your sleep woes? Both benzodiazepines and z-drugs are addictive and cause tolerance – a situation in which the body gets used to the drug and needs higher doses to achieve the same effect. They are addictive tablets, so if used for longer than a few weeks, people end up taking drugs that are no longer particularly effective at the prescibed dose but are difficult to stop due to dependence. These drugs can also cause dizziness and drowsiness the following day, especially in older people, increasing the risk of accidents and falls and potentially serious consequences, such as hip fractures. Additionally, they can cause impaired thinking and slow down reaction times, which may have an impact on driving or operating machinery. Sleeping tablets can occasionally cause a form of sleepwalking in which people get up in the night and may undertake dangerous activities, such as driving, with no memory the next day of what they have done. Z-drugs can also cause psychiatric symptoms, including confusion, hallucinations and nightmares.

Where z-drugs seem to be better than other sleeping tablets is that they do not seem to disturb the normal sleep architecture. Benzodiazepines reduce the amount of time spent in deep slow-wave sleep, and so people do not wake up feeling as refreshed. Z-drugs do not seem to have this effect.

A most alarming effect of taking sleeping tablets was discovered in a study published in 2012. Patients who were prescribed sleeping tablets had a substantially higher death rate compared with those not prescribed these drugs. This was a study in the USA involving over 30,000 patients over 30 months. Those patients taking fewer than 18 doses of sleeping pills in a year had three and a half times the death rate compared to patients not taking any sleeping pills, while for those taking over 132 doses the death rate was five times higher. This does not prove that the sleeping pills caused the increased deaths, but for a treatment that has only small benefits it is another important consideration.

## People present with sleeping disorders because of underlying conditions

So do sleeping tablets have a role in treatment? We know that they do work in the short term and have a useful role in treating an acute situation, such as following bereavement, in which case it is humane to prescribe them. For the majority of people for whom sleeping disorders are a chronic issue, however, sleeping tablets are far less beneficial. For most of these people, there are underlying issues causing the sleep disorders; these include stress and worries, mental health conditions, such as anxiety or depression, and physical disorders, including joint pain or neurological disease. Tackling these underlying issues with, for example, psychological treatments produces far better effects than medication. Unfortunately, people who have taken sleeping tablets for many years may feel that their sleeping disorders are beyond their own control.

## Summary

Tablets, potions and medicines have been used for a long time to deal with sleep issues. Despite their obvious success, their side effects and dependency have made doctors reluctant to prescribe them. They may prescribe some of the safer drugs for a very short period of time, to help you over a particularly acute phase. Treatment of any underlying conditions may be the approach that is needed.

## Top tips

1 Use either prescribed or over-the-counter medication reluctantly, only when all alternative strategies have not worked.
2 Only take medication for a very short period of time.
3 Look at other medical causes of poor sleep, such as pain or psychological disorders.

# 40

# 'When I've caught up on my sleep I can sort out the clutter'

I have just returned from my holidays. Feeling jet-lagged, my body is just getting used to the time change and I haven't had time to unpack yet. My bedroom is full of open cases with clothes spilling out, waiting to be washed or folded and put away, bags of toothpaste and deodorant. Once I've had a good sleep and don't feel so tired, I'll get around to sorting it all out. At least that is the plan. Does this sound familiar?

### Research shows clutter is associated with worse sleep

In a study presented at the Annual Meeting of the Associated Professional Sleep Societies, in Seattle in 2015, people had been questioned about their hoarding behaviour, using a clutter and hoarding rating scale. Hoarding is when people keep items that they do not need and experience distress with even the thought of getting rid of them. The participants were also asked about their sleep habits, using a questionnaire called the Pittsburgh Sleep Quality Index. This index is an internationally recognized way of assessing the quality and quantity of sleep. It ranges from 0, which is the best sleep, to 21, which is the worst. The scale records how long you sleep for, how tired you feel during the day, the use of medication and whether or not you snore.

Those who were more at risk of hoarding reported more difficulty sleeping than the tidier participants. They took longer to fall asleep, had more disturbed sleep and, as a result, were more tired during the day. The lack of sleep can also result in an increase in depression and anxiety. Hoarders typically have difficulties with decision-making, and the poor sleep can make this even worse.

You have probably seen programmes on the television about hoarders; people who can't throw anything away. Some have piles of newspapers, every one they have ever bought; others have every toy their children ever had and they feel unable to part with any of them. Ultimately, these people, who struggle so much with their belongings, need psychological support and help. There is so often a clear big life event, with parents or children, that leads to this behaviour.

## How is this relevant to me?

You are probably thinking, 'Well, I'm not the tidiest person in the world, but I am a long way from being classified as a hoarder' and you're probably right. This is not only about those who hoard at a level that would have television crews knocking at their door, however. It is about people who simply have too much clutter. The study mentioned above wasn't looking at people who were as extreme as the examples seen on television. Rather, it looked at whether or not people were at risk of hoarding. Having clutter in your bedroom is probably enough to disrupt your sleep. It isn't uncommon that people climb over piles of washing on the floor, skirting around boxes of old books to reach their bed for sleep.

A cluttered room will affect you consciously or unconsciously and stop you from fully relaxing overnight. It may create feelings of guilt or frustration or make you feel anxious about getting things tidy. While you may be able to ignore the mess because it's been there for a long time, subconsciously the brain wants to get things straight. This mental activity impedes full relaxation. Also, it doesn't just affect the time you are trying to get to sleep; it will probably also cause you to wake in the night as your mind is alive with clutter. As well as dealing with physical clutter, you also need to think about mental clutter. Are you thinking about your work, your family, your friends? This mental clutter may be an extension of your physical clutter.

## Make your bedroom tidy

Remember how your mum used to nag you to tidy your room? I now do this with my kids – so frustrating, but a serious first-world problem. Maybe she was right all along. Make your environment, particularly your bedroom, clean and tidy. This should even include the smell. For some, a clean and tidy bedroom is their haven. You could then think about the clutter in your entire house and garden, your car, your life.

Try to organize your rooms, particularly your bedroom, for their intended purpose. Your bedroom is for sleeping in. There is no need to have a pile of books, a set of crockery, stationery. Think carefully about this, and take pride and enjoyment in organizing your rooms. Think with joy about the people you can help by giving away surplus items to friends or family, and the charities that will benefit from your donations. De-clutter and bring happiness to yourself and others.

## Summary

Even small amounts of physical clutter in your environment may be having an impact on your sleep. Your physical environment may leak into your thoughts and feelings, creating a barrier to restful sleep. Look at strategies for dealing with this, and try to enjoy the process of becoming clutter-free.

## Top tips

1 Assign a role to each of the rooms in your house. Make sure items that you need are in the right place.
2 Give away anything you do not need. Be as ruthless as you can be.
3 Enjoy the feelings of positivity in your role in helping other people.

# Conclusion: how to sleep better

As you have seen from the preceding 40 chapters, there are many, many myths around sleep. Looking at these myths is a fascinating journey through the human psyche, the environment, our hopes and sometimes quite literally our dreams. Some of these ideas have a basis in truth, some of them may be quite helpful, but many are unfortunately misleading or possibly harmful.

When I first discussed the idea for this book with friends and colleagues, they were a little dismissive. They had not appreciated the sheer volume of mythology that surrounds sleeping, leading to both good and bad outcomes. Once I had accumulated a number of these stories, I started to discuss the ideas and – this was a shock for me – so many people had more stories to tell, many of which are in these pages.

These ideas were helpful as I looked at the ways to help you sleep better. This book has been about empowerment, not prescription. You can feel that your knowledge is powerful – your understanding of your body, of the way it works and how sleep operates. Allow yourself to take a while to consider your world, your ideas, your thoughts, your behaviours.

Then make a plan. I am keen on plans. You may like to write a list (like my wife), you may be less systematic (like me). Either way, formulate a plan, think carefully and go for it. Remember, too, that your age is no barrier to good sleep, although as Chapter 37 described, your sleep patterns are likely to change as you get older and your body changes.

When you examine your sleep truthfully, you may realize some of the factors that may be harming your sleep and your well-being. Some of what you do may be helpful. A straightforward positive first step could be to work out how you sleep. Chapter 1 considered the use of a sleep diary. It is a very good idea to do this at different times, as you attempt to sleep better. Filling in a sleep diary for a couple of weeks should give you an idea of how you are sleeping at the moment. You could also try using a device or app for your smartphone to give a more objective understanding of your sleep (see Chapter 21).

As you examine your sleep diary, can you see that you are accruing a sleep debt? Is your social life, your family life or your work life making you sleep less? Can you repay the debt swiftly? Chapter 31 discussed this, and advised that if you can avoid getting into a debt in the first place, this prevention is far better than a repayment. If this is not possible, however, then try to pay the debt back as soon as you can.

You should also try to work out how sleepy you are during the day and how long it takes you to fall asleep. Chapter 3 looked at this, using the method with the spoon. You could also investigate this using the technology on your smartphone.

## Consider your well-being

Let's deal with the first, and an essential, part of sleeping better: your psychology, your mental state, the emotions you feel and the actions you take. You must take time to consider these things. Are your feelings appropriate for your situation? Are you as good as you can be? Be truthful with yourself – you may have to accept some difficult realities.

Sometimes, regardless of any other advice or help, you must deal with your mental health issues first, which will help you to sleep better. I have met many people who are struggling with serious issues that are wreaking havoc with their slumber. My advice must be to seek some help from either your local general practitioner or a psychologist.

It is important to approach these strategies with the right mindset. For example, you should feel positive that what you are trying will work; you are going to give it your best shot. Remember, your social and personal circumstances may play a role in helping – or hindering – you in getting a better night's sleep, as Chapter 33 discussed. A difficult issue may be if you regularly take medication to help your sleep. The medical advice is to use these only when you have really tried everything else – and then only for a short period of time, for the reasons given in Chapter 39.

The next issue is to work out whether or not you have a serious sleep disorder. There are many – in excess of 70 – sleep disorders, ranging from breathing issues such as sleep apnoea (looked at in Chapter 35), through to much rarer disorders such as sleepwalking (Chapter 11). If you feel you may have a specific disorder, it is important that you seek a medical opinion. A doctor will be able to make an objective assessment: that is his or her job. You should take seriously any advice or intervention offered. Also, when you do get some advice or help, please try following it for a decent length of time to give it a chance to work; don't reject it after a short try. My wife, who is a general practitioner, wishes she could prescribe 'time'; it is a healer.

## Your time management

This is a key component of sleep management. Your time is governed, in part, by your body clock, known as your circadian rhythm. As shown in Chapter 15, your rhythm is directed by the things going on in your environment. Much of this is under your control, in things such as keeping a regularity to your day. Try to do things in a routine way, such as eating breakfast, lunch and evening meal the same time each day (covered in Chapter 32). Set your alarm clock to the same time each day, even weekends if you feel up to it.

When you have a day when you wake feeling refreshed and not excessively sleepy through the day, that is the right amount of sleep for you. Don't allow yourself to be convinced by others that there is a right amount of sleep, as discussed in Chapters 1 and 16. It doesn't matter what your friends do or tell you; only you can know what is right for you. Remember that one of the most harmful myths is the 8-hour sleep one.

In addition to this, sleeping is not a competition. Your sleep will be different from that of your bed partner, your friends or your children. As Chapter 24 reinforced, these differences are not anything to worry about: they are completely normal.

If you wake up in the middle of the night, don't panic and don't fight it. It is common for people to be distressed by this, leading to further difficulty sleeping. Chapter 12 looked at the need to be accepting of waking in the night. If you do wake, remain calm; accept this wakening. Try not to turn on any lights; consider some calm breathing exercises. Given time, you should find that you have fallen asleep again.

Think carefully about using an alarm to wake up. Do you feel tired every morning? This may mean you simply need to go to bed earlier. Try bringing your bedtime forward gradually until you reach a point at which you are able to feel awake when your alarm goes off, as discussed in Chapter 4. If you use your snooze button, then do you go back to sleep or lie quietly waiting for the day? If the former, you need to try to change that plan. Does your alarm clock gently light up to help wake you? Consider one of these.

Have you worked out your sleep pattern? Do you naturally awaken in the night? Try to embrace this if you feel it is incorrect. Chapter 6 discussed this at some length. Be careful, though, if you are trying to create more time in your day by varying your sleep patterns. Finally, in time management, have a think about what you are trying to achieve in your day. Chapter 30 looked at this, and you might want to reframe the activities you conduct. It may be that a more efficient you could achieve far more than the you who had less sleep.

## Your environment

The impact of your environment on your sleep is often underestimated. Check the darkness of your bedroom during the middle of the day by closing curtains and blinds fully, so you can see and then eliminate any sources of light that might creep in at dawn and wake you (buy blackout blinds if necessary). This should allow your body to know it is time for sleep.

Don't have a television in your bedroom if you can have it in an alternative location, as discussed in Chapter 13. Think about dimmer switches for your bedroom lighting. Try not to use devices at bedtime, or near bedtime, that project blue light – Chapters 27 and 38 showed how this has an impact. Try reading a book, preferably not a backlit tablet or computer.

Look at the temperature of your bedroom, as advised in Chapter 18. You may want to buy a simple room thermometer and make sure the temperature falls between 16 and 20 °C (61–68 °F). This should be all year round, which may entail some heating during the winter and the use of cooling fans during the summer.

Finally, think about the clutter in your world, as touched on in Chapter 40. This can mean your house, your bedroom, your office, your car. Try to be ruthless with things that you don't need but take up room. This is similar to mental clutter, which you also could tackle.

## Your lifestyle

Your lifestyle is incredibly important to your well-being and sleep. Chapter 10 discussed the need to be aware of your caffeine intake. It is found in many products and may be having an effect. Think about cutting out caffeine as far as you can for a few weeks, and then try the sleep diary again to see if the time you spend asleep improves. Be aware of alcoholic drinks – they may help you fall asleep, but does this improve the quality of your sleep? Chapter 28 considered this and, after reading it, you might think about making a change in the amount and timing of your consumption of alcohol.

Think carefully about your sleep patterns and how these may affect your weight management. Chapter 2 looked at this and the need to try to avoid those vicious circles; it talked about maintaining your motivation for sticking with a sensible eating plan with regular exercise. Chapters 23 and 36 discussed types of food and their impact on your sleep. The person who understands this best is you; you will know what keeps you awake at night or wakes you with heartburn. Begin to manage your eating to make night-time more straightforward.

Exercise can generally be positive for your sleep, but as pointed out in Chapter 25, be aware that high-intensity exercise close to bedtime may hinder falling asleep. The advice is to finish moderate levels of exercise around 3 hours before your normal bedtime.

## Active approaches to sleeping better

When you have tried all these methods, consider using some of these techniques:

1 Try some of the behavioural control techniques. Associate your bed with sleep, and sleep only.

2 Have a go at using a muscle-relaxation technique, such as the one described in Chapter 29.

3 Mindfulness: try a mindfulness class, or one for some other form of meditation. To give this the best chance, you will need to spend some time working on it. You could have a go at these techniques at home, now. Chapter 7 gives some hints and techniques you could try. Shane recommends concentrating on your breathing first, feeling the cool air across your nostrils, flowing into your lungs. Concentrating on this simple activity often allows thoughts to take far less precedence. Let them drift away.

4 Should you either take, or stop taking, a nap? As discussed in Chapters 17 and 19, a scheduled nap may make you more productive. This policy is gradually being adopted by some employers. Could this help you? As a guide, keep any nap you do take to under 20 minutes. Any more and you may wake up feeling groggy.

5 Go outside during the day; take some sunshine. This will help you to entrain your body clock so it knows where it is. Consider moderate exercise in the daytime, outside in the light.

We have gone through a whole series of things that you can do, you need to think about, you might worry about, but most of all, believe in yourself. You can do it.

# Useful addresses and websites

**British Sleep Society**
c/o EBS
City Wharf
Davidson Road
Lichfield WS14 9DZ
Tel.: 01543 442156
Email: admin@sleepsociety.org.uk
Website: www.sleepsociety.org.uk

**Children's Sleep Charity**
St Catherine's House
Woodfield Park
Tickhill Road
Doncaster DN4 8QP
Tel.: 01302 751416
Email: info@thechildrenssleepcharity.org.uk
Website: www.thechildrenssleepcharity.org.uk

**Sleep Apnoea Trust**
PO Box 60
Chinnor OX39 4XE
Tel.: 0800 025 3500
Email: Info@sleep-apnoea-trust.org
Website: www.sleep-apnoea-trust.org

**Some websites you might find useful**
Mindfulness-based stress reduction: www.umassmed.edu/cfm
Acceptance and commitment therapy (ACT):
   https://contextualscience.org/act
Buddhism and science: www.mindandlife.org
Thich Nhat Hanh and Buddhist links: www.iamhome.org
Meditation: http://whatmeditationreallyis.com

# Further reading

Cantopher, T. (2014) *Beating Insomnia*. London: Sheldon Press.

Carrell, S. E., Maghakian, T. and West, J. E. (2011) 'A's from zzzz's? The causal effect of school start time on the academic achievement of adolescents', *American Economic Journal: Economic Policy* 3(3): 62–81.

Dalai Lama and Cutler, H. (1998) *The Art of Happiness: A handbook for living.* New York: Riverhead.

Ebrahim, I. O., Shapiro, C. M., Williams, A. J. and Fenwick, P. B. (2013) 'Alcohol and sleep I: Effects on normal sleep', *Alcoholism: Clinical and Experimental Research* 37(4): 539–49.

Ekirch, R. (2005) *At Day's Close: Night in times past.* London: Norton.

Goleman, D. (2003) *Destructive Emotions: How can we overcome them?* New York: Bantam/Dell.

Gunaratana, B. (2002) *Mindfulness in Plain English.* Somerville, MA: Wisdom Publications.

Kabat-Zinn, J. (2005) *Coming to Our Senses: Healing ourselves and the world through mindfulness.* New York: Bantam.

Lovett, R. (2005) 'Coffee: The demon drink?', *New Scientist* 24: 2518–22.

# Index